W9-BPM-481

Probiotic Foods for Good Health

Yogurt, Sauerkraut, and Other Beneficial Fermented Foods

Beatrice Trum Hunter

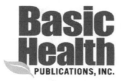

Basic Health
PUBLICATIONS, INC.

The information contained in this book is based upon the research and personal and professional experiences of the author. It is not intended as a substitute for consulting with your physician or other healthcare provider. Any attempt to diagnose and treat an illness should be done under the direction of a healthcare professional.

The publisher does not advocate the use of any particular healthcare protocol but believes the information in this book should be available to the public. The publisher and author are not responsible for any adverse effects or consequences resulting from the use of the suggestions, preparations, or procedures discussed in this book. Should the reader have any questions concerning the appropriateness of any procedures or preparation mentioned, the author and the publisher strongly suggest consulting a professional healthcare advisor.

Basic Health Publications, Inc.
28812 Top of the World Drive
Laguna Beach, CA 92651
949-715-7327 • www.basichealthpub.com

Library of Congress Cataloging-in-Publication Data

Hunter, Beatrice Trum.
  Probiotic foods for good health : yogurt, sauerkraut, and other beneficial fermented foods / Beatrice Trum Hunter.
     p. cm.
   Includes index.
   ISBN 978-1-59120-217-2
   1. Probiotics. 2. Fermented foods—Health aspects. I. Title.

RM666.P835H86   2008
613.2'6—dc22
                                                    2008031219

Copyright © 2008 Beatrice Trum Hunter

All rights reserved. No part of this book may be reproduced, stored in a retrieval system, or transmitted by any means, electronic, mechanical, photocopying, recording, or other-wise, without written permission from the author.

Editor: Cheryl Hirsch
Typesetting/Book design: Gary A. Rosenberg
Cover design: Mike Stromberg

Printed in the United States of America

10   9   8   7   6   5   4   3   2   1

To Cheryl Hirsch and Ruth Mary Pollack
with heartfelt appreciation

Contents

Part Three
Fermented Non-Dairy Foods

Appendices

Introduction

Many people seem to be obsessed with a desire to maintain a germ-free environment. It may come as a shock for them to learn that the human intestinal tract is home to an estimated 100 trillion bacteria. This staggering number includes many beneficial microbes that help keep the body healthy by fending off pathogenic ones that otherwise might colonize in the intestinal tract.

The state of good health or disease can be compared to the metaphor of warfare: a constant battle is waged between the forces of good (the beneficial microbes) and the forces of evil (the pathogenic microbes). Both armies engage in continuous skirmishes against each other, in living environments of soils; in and on plants, including food and feed crops; and in animals, including livestock and ourselves. The beneficial microbes attempt to prevent the foodborne pathogens from establishing "beachheads" by adherence in our guts, where they thrive, proliferate, and inflict harm. If the beneficial microbes are overwhelmed, the pathogenic ones win battles by causing infections and diseases. Within the context of living organisms, the beneficial microbes experience the ravages of war. Fortunately, the beneficial organisms have strategic "weapons" to rout, immobilize, and defeat the enemy. These weapons are *probiotics.*

All too frequently, the concept of probiotics is limited to probiotic dietary supplements, to the exclusion of the time-honored probiotic foods. In this book, I will emphasize probiotic foods. Probiotic dietary supplements may offer benefits as medical adjuvants, but the day-by-day consumption of foods with probiotic benefits are the ones that deserve primary consideration. As with other dietary supplements, the probiotics should not replace foods, but serve as adjuncts for intestinal health. (To learn more about probiotic supplements, see Appendix A on page 153.)

FORMER DISMISSAL OF PROBIOTIC FOODS

For too many years, the U.S. Department of Agriculture (USDA) denied the probiotic value of yogurt. In its 1965 Yearbook, *Consumers All*, the USDA discussed yogurt in a section titled "Food Quackery." The agency assured consumers that "yogurt has no food or health values other than those present in the kind of milk from which it is made." This pronouncement was ludicrous, even at the time when it was made. The agency chose to ignore evidence of the additional values developed in fermented milk: its bactericidal activity against foodborne pathogens; its ability to synthesize certain vitamins; its role in alleviating many gastrointestinal distresses and other health disorders; its usefulness in relieving antibiotic-induced effects; and its beneficial role for lactose-intolerant individuals.

Over the years, research conducted by the USDA's own Agricultural Research Service (ARS), as well as research conducted elsewhere, established evidence that yogurt has food and health values beyond those present in the milk from which it is made. The additional benefits are due to the probiotics in the fermented milk. Similarly, sauerkraut has values beyond cabbage, and other fermented foods have values beyond their original state.

DEFINING PROBIOTICS

As interest in probiotics has grown, experts have debated how to define probiotics specifically, according to the National Center for Complementary and Alternative Medicine (NCCAM) at the National Institutes of Health (NIH). One widely used definition, developed by the United Nations Food and Agricultural Organization/World Health Organization (FAO/WHO), designates probiotics as:

> . . . live microorganisms, which, when administered in adequate amounts, confer a health benefit on the host.

Other definitions are more inclusive. R. Havenaar and J. H. J. Huis in't Veld, in *The Lactic Acid in Health and Disease* (Elsevier, 1992), suggest probiotics are:

> . . . a viable mono- or mixed culture of microorganisms which, when applied to animals or man, beneficially affect the host by improving the

properties of the indigenous microbiota [microflora in the digestive tract].

G. Reuter, in "Present and Future Probiotics in Germany and in Central Europe," (*Biosci Microflora*, 1997) offers this definition:

. . . a microbial preparation which contains live and/or dead cells, including their metabolites [byproducts], which is intended to improve the microbial or enzymatic balance at mucosal surfaces or to stimulate immune mechanism.

R. Fuller, in "Probiotics in Man and Animals" (*J Appl Bacteriol*, 1989), proposes that probiotics are:

. . . a live microbial food supplement which beneficially affects the host animal by improving its intestinal microbial balance.

R. B. Parker, in "Probiotics: The Other Half of the Antibiotic Story" (*Anim Nutr Health*, 1974), includes humans as well as other animals in food supplements that:

. . . have a beneficial effect on the host animal by affecting the gut microflora.

Live beneficial microorganisms promote a physiologic balance essential for good health in humans and other animals.

APPRECIATION AND UTILIZATION OF PROBIOTICS

To continue the war metaphor used earlier, the world seems to be overrun by pathogens. Each of us, in a volunteer army, should recognize the microbial allies that have evolved with, and support, our wellbeing. Unfortunately, the food processors, like a World War II fifth column, have infiltrated our ranks and undermined our health, by perverting the fermentation process. The food processors offer us yogurt-coated pretzels and frozen yogurts, chemically fermented soft drinks and alcoholic beverages, canned sauerkraut, and unfermented soy products, among others. We need to be on guard against these enemies within the camp, oust them, and strengthen the corps. We need to do constant battle with pathogens intent on our destruction, and allow the powerful forces of probiotics to secure and maintain the peace of health and wellbeing.

This book will demonstrate that fermented foods, such as yogurt and sauerkraut among others, help to maintain and restore good health. As the results of many human experiences through the centuries, the benefits of fermented foods have been recognized. Currently, fermented foods continue to be valued and used in traditional diets, but unfortunately they have been largely discarded in the Western diet.

There is no mention of fermented foods in the federal 2005 Dietary Guidelines for Healthy Americans, which provide advice about the foods and dietary habits that can promote health and reduce risk for major chronic disease, or in the numerous graphic versions of food pyramids. Rarely do Western physicians or nutritionists recommend fermented foods to patients. Nor are fermented foods included in dietary sheets given by dietitians to patients. The indexes of books by current writers on food and nutrition—people who are acknowledged as authorities in the field—fail to list any discussions of fermented foods. The ARS of the USDA has found many benefits of lactic acid bacteria (the principle agent responsible for fermentation) in its various research projects, but the agency rarely has translated the findings into practical applications for human health.

The time is long overdue to recognize something known, but forgotten: the health benefits of fermented foods. The recognition should encourage us to add health-promoting fermented foods to our daily diet.

PART ONE

Fermentation: A Venerable Tradition

CHAPTER 1

Probiotics: New Applications for Old Knowledge

At present, probiotics is not a familiar term to many people. It will become more familiar. Probiotics (meaning "for life") are foods that are cultured with live beneficial microorganisms. Digested in sufficient amounts, they can combat pathogenic microbes and bestow functional or health benefits. Probiotic foods are fermented foods. Perhaps the best recognized ones are yogurt and sauerkraut. Many more exist.

In recent years, the sales of probiotic supplements as well as probiotic foods have risen meteorically in the United States. By 2003, sales were nearly $13 million annually, with a spectacular 14 percent increase in yearly sales. In terms of importance in food-product formulations, probiotics rose from tenth place in 2000 to fifth place by 2005. The increased sales were stimulated by federal research.

NEW USES IN AGRICULTURE

Since 1996 governmental funding for agricultural applications of probiotic research has doubled annually. The U.S. Department of Agriculture's (USDA) Agricultural Research Service (ARS) has conducted studies with biopreservatives such as probiotic bacteria produced by lactic acid, bacteriocins, and bacteriophages. As a result, some farmers use probiotics to help boost disease resistance in crops, increase reproduction in farm animals, and increase milk and egg production. Such increases are achieved by better health of crops and animals, bestowed by the probiotics. However, the findings have not yet been applied to people.

NEW USES FOR FOOD SAFETY

Governmental agencies responsible for food safety, the food industry, and the consuming public are concerned about the alarming number of incidences of foodborne diseases causing illnesses and deaths, resulting from the consumption of raw or undercooked foods that are contaminated with various pathogenic microbes. The Centers for Disease Control and Prevention (CDC) estimate that some 76 million Americans experience foodborne illnesses every year. About 325,000 of them are so serious that they require hospitalization. Some 5,000 people die. Some critics charge that these numbers are *gross underestimations*. Many infected people do not seek medical attention. Those who do may be misdiagnosed. Also, many cases may go unreported. The reporting system is largely "passive," that is, voluntary rather than mandatory.

The list keeps growing of contaminated foods that have been responsible for outbreaks of foodborne illnesses and deaths. Among them, recently, are spinach, lettuce, mixed salad greens, green onions, endive, watercress, parsley, cabbage, sprouts of alfalfa, radish and mung beans, water chestnuts, carrots, tomatoes, melons, raspberries, strawberries, apple cider, carrot and orange juices, ground beef, chicken, turkey, fish, soft cheeses, egg salad, coleslaw, peanut butter, and almonds.

In attempts to prevent contamination of foods by pathogenic microbes, researchers have taken a fresh look at one of the powerful agents that prevents food spoilage: lactic acid bacteria, the principal agent responsible for fermentation.

One example of using lactic acid bacteria for food safety is with raw produce. In a search to find substitutes for the harsh chemical sanitizers used with raw fruits and vegetables, Alejandro Castillo at Texas A&M University at College Station, and his colleagues in Mexico, reported in the *Journal of Food Protection* (Sept 2007) about their success with lactic acid bacteria. The researchers intentionally exposed cantaloupe and bell peppers either to *Escherichia coli* 0157:H7 *(E. coli)* or *Salmonella typhimurium*. Both are virulent types of bacteria that contaminate foods. Then, the researchers sprayed a lactic acid solution on the produce for fifteen seconds. The treatment reduced dramatically the bacterial populations on the rough and crinkled rind of the cantaloupe by nearly 99.9 percent, and by slightly more on the smooth-surfaced bell pepper. Although we do not consume the rind of melons, there have been outbreaks of foodborne illness in individuals who had eaten melons. The rinds had not been washed, and were contaminated with pathogenic microbes. In cutting the melons, the knives had transferred the microbes to the interior edible portion.

Castillo and his colleagues also conducted experiments with animals. They reported that a 2 percent lactic acid spray was effective in sanitizing carcasses.

The Institute of Food Technology, in its publication *Food Technology* (Sept 1997), reported that use of lactic acid bacteria was effective in improving the safety of minimally processed fruits and vegetables.

Decades ago, researchers at Cornell University, had noted that a raw vegetable, washed in a vinegar solution, reduced the surface contamination of lead on raw produce. Vinegar is a product of fermentation. More recently, the *Journal of Food Protection* (May 2003) reported that washing apples in a vinegar solution resulted in a significant reduction of *Salmonella*.

There is growing recognition of the value of fermentative agents for the control of pathogens. This recognition offers a valuable tool in the large issue of food safety. In addition, another feature makes the fermentation process attractive to the food industry.

NEW USES IN FOOD-PRODUCT DEVELOPMENT

In recent years, there has been a growing interest in so-called functional foods. These are foods to which novel or unique ingredients are incorporated, purportedly for health benefits. Currently, federal statutory and regulatory provisions require that such added ingredients used in food formulations that bear health or structural function claims must be approved for their intended uses. Doubtless, among the new functional foods will be fermented products.

In Europe, consumers have embraced probiotic-fortified dairy products. In contrast, Americans have had a deep-rooted perception that all bacteria are "bad." According to Niklas Bjärum, sales and marketing director of Probi, a Swedish biotechnology company, American attitudes are changing, and Americans are coming to accept the idea that some bacteria can be beneficial. Bjärum remarked in 2007 that "The United States market has been a sleeping beauty. But it's a question of when it wakes up to probiotics—not if—and I think that time is now."

The functional food frenzy already has begun. "Nutritionally enhanced" yogurt is regarded as a functional food. Many more will follow. At a time when "healthy foods," "fortified foods," and "enriched foods" appeal to a health-conscious public, fermented foods will come to be regarded by the food industry as a profitable extension of new food-product development. Within the categories of acceptable claims for health or structure, food processors are touting product benefits to the immune system, the digestive tract, and the genitourinary tract, and others for the alleviation of specific health disorders.

NEW USES AS ANTIBIOTIC RESISTANCE INCREASES

The rising incidence of pathogenic contamination in the food supply results from many factors, including a radical transformation of agriculture and the misuse, overuse, and growing ineffectiveness of antibiotics. The issue is only part of a larger one, concerning pathogenic contamination of the environment.

Antimicrobials have been available for a long time. But the growing problem of environmental contamination has generated a new industry. The goal is to make the environment germ free, an impossible task and an unwise objective. In attempting to make the environment germ free, both the beneficial as well as the pathogenic microorganisms are destroyed. Probiotics is a wiser choice, in using beneficial microorganisms to suppress and kill the pathogens. However, the trend favors use of antimicrobials.

Much effort is devoted to create "germ-free" environments. Many antimicrobial products are available. Alcohol-based products now substitute for thorough hand-washing with soap and hot water. Antimicrobials are used to treat children's toys, furniture, fabrics, and a wide array of other consumer goods. Ironically, some of the very substances used for this purpose are suspect.

The prevalent hospital-induced infections from *Staphylococcus aureus* ("staph infection") has led to ongoing research to produce antimicrobials intended for hospital airducts, walls, ceilings, floors, railings, doors and doorknobs. The research extends to appliances inserted into the body, such as artery-opening stents, and to prosthetic body parts, such as artificial limbs.

Many uses would extend to public places. For example, the aircraft manufacturer Boeing has expressed interest in coating surfaces in its planes touched by passengers, such as hard surfaces and fabrics. Other coatings are intended to kill viruses (for example, the influenza virus) on contact. Such substances also may be added to paints brushed or sprayed onto surfaces.

These attempts to achieve germ-free environments result in unintended consequences. The "hygiene hypothesis" demonstrates that we need some exposure to germs in order to develop mechanisms and substances in our bodies that are capable of resisting infections. It has been observed, for example, that children who grow up on farms, exposed to farm animals, are at lower risk of infections than are urban children sheltered in highly antiseptic environments. This is not to condemn cleanliness, but rather to recognize the value of a strong immune system that helps to buffer the body from assaults by pathogens. Either infections may not occur, or they may be mild and allow the body to recuperate quickly. The immune system can be kept healthy and strong by probiotics.

CHAPTER 2

Fermentation: An Old and Widespread Practice

The fermentation of foods and beverages was a chance discovery in prehistoric times. The transformation of wild and cultivated grains, fruits, and berries to beer, wine, and other foods, must have seemed miraculous. The mysterious process may have inspired later alchemists, who sought to transmute base metals such as lead, into noble ones such as gold.

BENEFICIAL MICROORGANISMS INVOLVED IN FERMENTATION

The fermentation of foods and beverages has been practiced nearly worldwide. Numerous types of wild yeasts, bacteria, and fungi (molds) have succeeded in creating a variety of fermented products. Fermentation of vegetables converts cabbage to sauerkraut, cucumbers to pickles, and other vegetable medleys to kimchi. Fermented grains, as just mentioned, made possible the creation of beer, and of bread leavened with sourdough or yeast. Fermented fruit such as grapes or berries transformed them into wines and distilled alcoholic beverages. Fermented honey turned to mead (honey wine). Fermented legumes such as soybeans, chickpeas, lentils, grams, and peanuts were converted into an array of new products, including tempeh, miso, *sufu*, and *idli*. Fermented milk produced a variety of dairy foods, including yogurt, kefir, buttermilk, and cheeses, among others. Even now, fermentation is used in processing the leaves of tea, the beans of coffee, and the pods of cocoa and vanilla.

Fermentation involves the growth of beneficial microorganisms that are capable of changing the original characteristics of foods. The principal ones are acids, especially lactic acid, which lower the pH of a food (a measure of its acidity or alkalinity) to such an extent that pathogenic

13

microbes are unable to thrive and multiply. The desirable microorganisms produce other chemicals as well, and these, too, are thought to have an inhibitory effect on the pathogens. (For detailed descriptions of these beneficial microorganisms, see Chapter 11.)

A wide variety of beneficial microorganisms are responsible for fermentation. Yeasts convert carbohydrates into alcohol. Fungi and bacteria create highly flavored hard cheeses. Bacteria produce lactic acid in cheddar cheese, pickles, and salami. A starter culture, such as used in yogurt, encourages rapid growth of the desirable microorganisms. Naturally present flora encourage the growth of desirable microorganisms in sauerkraut, tea, coffee, and cocoa. Fermentation, in addition to its role in preservation, produces new flavors and textural changes, as witnessed in the conversion of cabbage to sauerkraut and grapes to wine.

Salt is an important ingredient in food fermentation. The degree of concentration of added salt influences the type of microorganisms that will predominate. For example, the salt added to shredded raw cabbage encourages lactic acid bacteria to ferment the cabbage and convert the vegetable to sauerkraut. Olives and cucumbers are prepared in a similar way by salt brining. Acetic acid (vinegar), another fermentation agent, may be added to assist in preventing the growth of pathogenic microbes.

EARLY FERMENTATION METHODS

At different times and in different places, various techniques have been used to break down the starch in grains such as barley, millet, wheat, or corn. The starch in the grain, broken down to glucose (a sugar), supports the growth of yeasts.

Perhaps the oldest method used was malting. The grain was moistened so that it could germinate. After a few days, the germinated grain generated enzymes that broke down the starch into glucose. The malting of grain was practiced early in beer making, both in Egypt and Babylon, before the third millennium BC. Beer was brewed with malted wheat or barley. In Egypt, the malted grain was preserved by baking it into a dried flat bread. Then, at a later time, when the beer was being made, the malted grain was revived by soaking the dry bread in water. The arts of brewing beer and making bread are intertwined.

In Peru, before the arrival of the Conquistadors, the Incas used another technique to break down the starch in grain. They prepared a fermented drink known as *chicha*, by having humans chew on ground corn. The enzymes in the saliva helped to break down the starch. (See the inset below to learn more about this practice by other cultures.)

Salivary Enzymes as Fermentative Aids

Girolamo Benzoni, in his sixteenth-century book *History of the New World*, reported on his observations of the technique used by the Incas to make a fermented drink called *chicha*. People would chew on the ground corn to break down the starch. Today, chicha is still made, but the old technique has been replaced, thanks to the modern science of enzymology, which plays an important role in food processing.

In some cultures, even today, caregivers chew on food and predigest it before offering it to infants. The adults' saliva helps make the food easier to digest. Humans may have developed this practice after observing parent birds regurgitate food and stuff it into the chicks' anticipatory beaks.

Honeybees, too, use enzymes to produce honey. The foraging bees gather nectar and mix it with enzymes in their stomach-like honey sacs to digest the nectar before passing it to the bees in the hive. The house bees reduce the moisture content of the mixture by ingesting and regurgitating before depositing drops of the mixture into the honeycomb cells.

The Innuits learned to use salivary enzymes for another purpose. By chewing on raw animal hides, they could soften the hides before further processing to make the hides into clothing.

In Asia, still another technique was employed to break down starch. *Aspergillus oryzae*, a mold, secretes an enzyme capable of digesting the starch in rice. The mold is known as koji. It has been used for years to prepare rice for fermentation into the rice wine, sake.

Many fermentation techniques evolved. Some probably resulted from trial and error; others, by keen observations. Whether by early chance contamination of food with wild yeasts, fungi, or bacteria in the air, or later by controlled inoculation of specific strains of microorganisms, the process of fermentation has bestowed numerous benefits.

CHAPTER 3

Fermented Foods and Beverages Around the Globe

The nearly universal practice of fermenting foods and beverages in traditional diets attests to their recognized values. Through trial and error, and keen observation, fermentation was recognized as a way of preserving foods and beverages for future use. Thus, in times of plenty, fermented foods were hedges against lean times. In regions of seasonal changes, crops grown and gathered in warm weather would still be available for consumption later in cold weather. People found that fermented foods and beverages added variety to the diet, with different and agreeable flavors. They noted special healthful features from these foods. For these various attributes and more, fermented foods and beverages became part of traditional diets around the world.

AFRICA

The Sudanese people may head the list as consumers of fermented foods and beverages. It is reported that people in the Sudan consume fermented products that include:

- ten different types of leavened breads

- ten different types of fermented porridge

- nine special fermented foods

- seven different types of fermented dairy sauces

- four different types of fermented meat sauces

- five different types of fermented fish sauces

- five different types of fermented substitute flavors from animal-based sources

- thirteen different types of beer
- five different types of wine
- one type of mead

Other Africans also consume a variety of fermented foods and beverages. Home-brewed beers are staples in the African diet. They are an important source of vitamin B. Also, the iron pots used for brewing contribute some dietary iron to the beers. Although this form of iron is not well absorbed, it does add some iron to diets that are low in iron-rich foods such as meat.

In South Africa, sorghum beer is made from fermented sorghum. At times, some corn is added to the sorghum. The beer is fermented by yeasts and bacteria.

In Zaire, fermentation of manioc root (also called cassava) cultured by yeasts, fungi, and bacteria, is used to make beer.

In West Africa, especially in Nigeria, *dawadawa* is made into balls from fermented millet. Sometimes it is made by fermenting the African locust bean, a legume. The products are fermented by yeasts and bacteria. Also in West Africa, *gari* is made from fermented cassava, and *ogi* from corn, fermented by bacteria and fungi, and then lightly toasted or fried. In Ghana, *banku* is a product made from fermented corn and cassava, and leavened by yeasts and bacteria. In Nigeria, *burukutu,* a popular alcoholic beverage, is a product made from fermented sorghum and cassava.

In East Africa, especially in Sudan, *nyufu* is made from dried and fermented tofu. Also in Sudan, *merissa* is made from fermented sorghum. In Ethiopia, a very large flat bread, known as *enjera* (or *injera*) is made by fermenting the tiny black grain, teff. Sometimes corn, wheat, or barley is added to the teff.

Kenkey is an African maize (corn) dumpling. It is fermented by yeasts, bacteria, and fungi.

ASIA

India is home to many fermented foods. In East India, *taotjo* is made from fermented soybeans and wheat, or rice. In South India, a fermented press cake made from peanuts is known as *ontjom*. *Papadam, waries,* and *dosai* are all made from black gram, a legume, and turned into crisp savory pancakes. They are fermented by yeasts and bacteria. *Khaman* is made from Bengal gram, and idli, a small cake, from black gram or rice. Both products are fermented by yeasts and bacteria. *Nan*, a flat bread, is a wheat product, fermented by yeasts. *Torani*, a sweet syrup, is made from fermented rice, and *kanji*, an alcoholic beverage, from fermented rice and carrots. *Dhoka* is made from wheat and/or legumes, fermented by yeasts and bacteria. *Jalabies* found in Nepal, India, and Pakistan, is made from fermented wheat flour.

Throughout Asia, fermented foods are common. *Ang-kak*, based on rice, is fermented by fungi. Soy sauce is common throughout the region. It is made from soybeans, or soybeans and wheat, and is fermented by fungi, yeasts, and bacteria. In Indonesia, *oncom* is a peanut press cake (mentioned earlier as *ontjom* in South India). *Bonkrek* is a coconut press cake. Widely used tempeh is made from soybeans, fermented by fungi. *Taupe* is made from cassava or rice. *Kecap*, a sweet soy sauce, is made from soybeans and wheat, and fermented by fungi, yeasts, and bacteria. In Sri Lanka, *hopper* is made from rice, and fermented with yeasts and bacteria. In Malaysia, shoyu, a type of soy sauce made from soybeans and wheat, is fermented by fungi, yeasts, and bacteria.

Japan has numerous fermented foods and beverages. *Katsuobushi* is fermented fish. The popular beverage, sake, is wine made from steamed fermented rice. Koji is made from fermented rice, and is consumed in China as well as in Japan. Miso paste is produced from soybeans in Japan, and from some cereal grains in China. Miso is fermented by fungi. *Hamanatto*, a savory soy nugget, is made from soybeans and wheat flour.

In China, *kaoling* is a liquor made by fermenting fruit or fruit juice. *Lao-cho* is produced in China and in Indonesia by fermenting rice by several fungi. *Meitanza* is a fermented soybean cake, made in Taiwan as well as on mainland China. *Minchin*, a condiment, is made from wheat gluten, and fermented by fungi. Sufu and *chee-fan* are fermented foods, both made from soybeans and whey curds. Sufu is used in Taiwan as well as on mainland China.

In Korea, *meju* is made by fermenting soybeans. A hot pepper bean paste is made into *kochujang*, fermented by fungi, yeasts, and bacteria.

PACIFIC RIM

In the Philippines, *burung hyphon* is made from shrimp and other seafood, fermented by yeasts. *Tao-si* is a product made from fermented soybeans and wheat flour. *Puto,* steamed bread made from rice, is fermented by fungi and bacteria.

In Hawaii, poi, a starch staple, is made from taro, and is fermented by fungi and bacteria. This food paste commonly accompanies meat, fish, or vegetables.

In New Zealand, the Maori people use *kaanga-kopuwai,* made from corn, and fermented by yeasts and bacteria.

EUROPE AND THE MIDEAST

Fermented milk beverages include *hangop* from Holland, *pumpermilch* from Germany, *bassmilch* from the Alpine region, *mezzoradu* from Switzerland, and *huslanka* and *udra* from the Carpathian Mountains area in central and eastern Europe.

Some fermented milk products have been made traditionally from raw milk, without heat treatment. They include *saya; piimä* (or *piimaa*), also known as *fiili biima* and *ropa,* from Finland; and *taette* or *t¢tte,* from the Scandinavian countries.

In Tadzhikistan, cheese curd is known as *chekka.* When it is salted and dried, it is called *kurut.*

Some groups of people combine yogurt with grains to bestow a long shelflife. This practice may have a very ancient origin. The *tayer* of the Jews was a product that was dried, kept in sacks, and then transported by camel, to be sold at distant villages.

Kishk is a Middle Eastern food mixture, consisting of leben (yogurt) and *burghul* (bulgur, which is parched cracked wheat). The mix is fermented, dried, powdered, and stored for future use. It is reconstituted with liquid.

The Turkish *tarhana* is made by mixing one part yogurt with two parts of coarse wheat flour that has been parboiled. Vegetables may be added. The mixture is allowed to ferment for several days. Then it is sun-dried and stored for future use. Iraqi *kushkik* (or *kushuk*) is prepared in a similar manner, without the addition of vegetables.

SOUTH AMERICA

The Latin American region is no stranger to fermented foods and beverages. Mexico produces pulque, a sourish beer made from fermented cactus. *Colonche,* a fermented drink, is made from prickly pears. *Tuba,* a coconut wine, is made from the sap of palm tree coconut, and fermented by yeasts. *Pozol*, corn dough or porridge, is fermented by fungi and bacteria.

In Peru, chicha is produced from corn. The drink is fermented by yeasts and bacteria.

In Ecuador, sierra rice is fermented by fungi and bacteria.

In Brazil, *jamin-bang* is made from corn. It is fermented by yeasts and bacteria.

NORTH AMERICA

Many of the fermented foods and beverages familiar to us originated elsewhere. Among the most popular are fermented dairy foods.

Many of the aged and fresh cheeses we enjoy had their beginnings in Europe. They are fermented with various *Penicillium* molds. Such mold-ripened cheeses include Brie, Camembert, Gorgonzola, Roquefort, and Stilton, among the aged cheeses, and cottage cheese, queso blanco, and farmer cheese, among the fresh ones. Other cultured dairy foods include soured milk, buttermilk, clabbered milk, clotted cream (Devonshire cream), and crème fraîche, as well as cultured butter.

Yogurt and other cultured milk drinks we enjoy had their beginnings mainly in the MidEast, with numerous variations in their names, spellings, and pronunciations in different locations. For example, it is *yoart* or *yoghourt* in Turkey, and elsewhere, it is *youghourt, yohurt, yahourth, jugurt,* and so forth. But others are less readily identifiable to us. To wit:

- Arabia: *leben*
- Armenia: *matsoon, mazum, mazun*
- Balkans: *turho, gisurt, yourt, yo-urt*
- Bohemia: *urgutrik*
- Bulgaria: *maya, kisselo mleko*
- Chile: *skuta*
- Egypt: *leben raib*
- India: *dahi, lassi, chas, matta*
- Iran: *mazun, madzoon, maslo, mast, airig, airag, yoghourt, choeneck*
- Sardinia, Corsica, and Sicily: *gioddon*
- Scandinavia: *gouddu*

- Syria: *laban*

- Turkestan: *busa*

Yogurt-type drinks include kefir from the Caucasus in Eurasia, made from cow's milk; *kumys* (or *kumiss*) from Russia, made from mare's milk; or *kuban* in southern Russia. In Norway, kefir is known as *kaelder* or *kyael meelk.*

These cultured dairy foods as well as each group of fermented grains, legumes, and vegetables will be discussed in detail later in the book.

THE PRACTICAL AND CULTURAL BENEFITS OF FERMENTED FOODS

The development of fermented foods and beverages globally allowed people to enjoy a wider variety of foods, and in different forms. The possibility of storing food for future use offered an opportunity to save surpluses in prosperous times as a buffer against lean times. Fermented foods allowed for more distant travel, with an assurance that food would be available during the journey. In turn, distant travel led to interchanges with other groups of people, and the possibility to exchange goods and ideas. Of utmost importance, fermented foods contributed to good health and food safety.

CHAPTER 4

Some Special Features
of Fermented Foods

Fermented foods led to cultural changes. In early times, fermented foods and beverages allowed for long distance travel on land or water, without any need to stop frequently to replenish supplies. The Vikings were Scandinavian seafaring traders, warriors, and raiders who also colonized wide areas of Europe from the late eighth to the eleventh century. They learned that during their long seafaring voyages, the crew would remain healthy even after the fresh food supply dwindled. Large casks of sauerkraut, taken aboard before departure, prevented the dreadful illness and death that we now know as scurvy. The Vikings may have been unaware that the vitamin C (ascorbic acid) content in the sauerkraut was the protective antiscorbutic substance, but they did recognize that the fermented food kept people healthy.

The British Navy was not so enlightened. Scurvy was regarded as the result of miasmas (poisonous air) or other uncontrollable forces. James Lind Senior, physician to the Royal Navy Hospital Haslar at Portsmouth, witnessed many cases of the disease. In 1795, Lind recommended that sailors be given lemon juice. The dread scourge disappeared from the British Navy. At times, limes were taken on board for the same purpose. As a result, British sailors became known as "limeys."

Through the years, people have come to appreciate some of the special features of fermented foods. They include affordability, energy efficiency, increased nutritional values, food safety, and food improvement.

LOW-COST AND ENERGY EFFICIENCY

In warm and humid climates, fermentation extends the life of foods by retarding spoilage. This benefit can be achieved at low cost, without the use of energy or any special equipment needed for other means of pre-

serving, such as cooking, pasteurizing, canning, freezing, drying, steriliz-
ing, irradiating, or using special techniques such as aseptic and vacuum
packagings.

In cooler climates, fermentation extends the range of dietary choices in
seasons when fresh produce is not always readily available.

In all climates, fermentation increases the nutrient density of the original foods.

THE EFFICIENCY OF FERMENTATION

Fermentation helps to salvage otherwise unusable or waste materials.
Fermentation converts them into usable foods for human consumption
(for example, windfall apples into cider), and feeds for animal consumption (for example, ensilage).

In some instances, the fermentation process increases certain nutrients
in the food. This is especially true for some of the vitamin B fractions,
achieved through vitamin synthesis.

Fermentation degrades protein foods into their amino acids. It achieves
this breakdown through proteolytic enzymes. This process spares the
body of the necessity to use energy to convert the proteins into a usable
form. The protein in fermented foods already has been partially digested.
The amino acids are bioavailable, and easily are absorbed directly into the
digestive system. Thus, fermented foods provide readily available nutrients efficiently to the body.

Some enzymes of microbial origin, which are essential for fermentation, are beneficial. For example, the strong proteolytic enzymes of *Rhizopus oligosporus* in the fermented soybean food, tempeh, brings about rapid
hydrolysis (breakdown by means of water) of protein to amino acids. In
miso, a fermented paste, the starch of the rice as well as the protein of the
soybean are hydrolyzed by the enzymes of *Aspergillus oryzae,* and become
more bioavailable.

THE ANTIBACTERIAL EFFECTS OF FERMENTATION

Production of an antibacterial compound by *R. oligosporus* and other strains
of the bacterium minimize infections from certain pathogenic microbes.
Also, the antibacterial compounds have beneficial growth-stimulating
effects on animals fed otherwise inadequate diets. The true nutritive value of fermented foods such as tempeh and others may be that antibiotics
are formed from the fermentative molds and, thus, offer safety benefits in

the resulting fermented foods. Also, the formed antibiotics can protect against reinfestation of harmful microbes.

Fermentation destroys toxic, undesirable, or antinutrient components that are present in some foods in a raw state. For example, raw soybeans contain naturally occurring antinutrients and toxins. These undesirable substances are reduced somewhat by sprouting or cooking the soybeans, but are deactivated by fermentation. (This topic is discussed in Chapter 15.)

FERMENTATION ENRICHES YOUR DIET

Fermentation can improve the appearance, texture, consistency, and flavor of foods. Often, such foods stimulate the appetite. And, in the examples of beer, wine, and distilled alcoholic beverages, these fermented liquids (in moderation) create pleasant exhilaration!

PART TWO

Yogurt and Other Fermented Milk Products

CHAPTER 5

Yogurt: An Ancient and Modern Food

Curdled milk products may have been discovered by Neolithic people shortly after they learned to milk animals. Milk, allowed to rest for a few hours in warm weather, would soon have curdled. Depending on which wild yeasts were floating in the air, the curds would be fine or coarse. The former would develop into a product similar to yogurt or other cultured milk drinks; the latter, into soft fresh cheese.

Eventually, humans discovered that they could precipitate curdling in milk by adding certain types of vegetable juices, or by pouring the milk into a leather pouch made from the stomach of a calf. The lining of its stomach contains an enzyme, rennin, which produces a curdling agent, rennet. No doubt, enzymes in the vegetable juices also were the agents responsible for curdling. People found that if they pressed the curds into basketry molds or perforated earthenware containers, the whey would drain out and the curds would form cheese.

Yogurt Factoids

It is believed that in the twelfth century yogurt was the mainstay in the diet of the hearty Mongolian nomads, who accompanied the warlord Genghis Khan in his invasion and occupation of most of Asia.

In the sixteenth century, Francis I, King of France, after a lifetime of debauchery, developed health problems. He summoned to his court a famous Turkish physician from Constantinople. The treatment consisted mainly of yogurt. The king recovered his health, and resumed his life of dissipation.

DISCOVERY OF PROBIOTIC'S BENEFICIAL EFFECTS

There has been a continuous, unbroken connection with yogurt and other cultured dairy foods from the distant past to the present. In modern times, one individual can be acknowledged as the father of probiotic research with yogurt. Professor Élie (Ilya) Metchnikoff, a Russian zoologist and bacteriologist by training, in 1904 became the second director of the Pasteur Institute in Paris. In 1908, Metchnikoff and Pasteur shared the prestigious Nobel Prize for their work in physiology and medicine.

Metchnikoff's major contributions were his pioneering efforts to explore the health benefits of yogurt. It was appropriate that a centennial celebration in recent years was held in his honor at a symposium on the clinical applications of probiotics in human health.

About 1898, a colleague of Metchnikoff's, Stamen Grigoroff, isolated the bacterium, *Lactobacillus bulgaricus*, from yogurt made in Bulgaria. Grigoroff reported to Metchnikoff that there were numerous centenarians living in Bulgaria who attributed their longevity to their daily habit of eating substantial amounts of homemade yogurt. Intrigued, Metchnikoff began to study this strain of lactic acid-producing bacterium for its possible therapeutic values. Convinced of the efficacy of the bacterium, Metchnikoff made it available commercially.

In the United States, the bacterium was used extensively to culture so-called Bulgarian buttermilk. However, the product was quite tart, and less palatable and less versatile in usage than yogurt.

In 1908, the same year that Metchnikoff became a Nobelist, two American scientists, Herter and Kendall, ran tests on monkeys with Bulgarian buttermilk. They disputed Metchnikoff's claim that the bacteria created lactic acid in the lower colon in sufficient amounts necessary to arrest any putrefaction and autointoxication. (Autointoxication is caused by wastes and toxins from the colon that seep into the bloodstream. This action poisons the body and can initiate chronic disease.) Controversy ensued and discouraged sales of Bulgarian buttermilk in the United States. In Europe, however, *L. bulgaricus* was used commonly to produce yogurt rather than buttermilk.

Metchnikoff's main interest became the role of beneficial microorganisms and their ability to protect human health. He conducted fruit fly experiments and found that the leukocytes (white blood cells) were antibodies, capable of destroying invading pathogenic microbes.

Metchnikoff became obsessed with the idea that there was a constant struggle waged between life-destroying and life-saving forces. He formulated a hypothesis about the "friendly" intestinal flora—a phrase that is still in use. He studied the diet of Bulgarians. Commonly, they ate quantities of homegrown vegetables and generous amounts of homemade yogurt. Metchnikoff attributed their longevity to their dietary habits. He found that, among Europeans, the Bulgarians had the greatest number of friendly intestinal flora in their digestive tracts.

By modern research standards, Metchnikoff's conclusions appear simplistic. He failed to examine numerous other factors that may have contributed to the health and longevity of the Bulgarians. Also, he was incorrect in believing that the beneficial bacteria, *L. bulgaricus*, which cultures yogurt, can be implanted in the intestine. In reality, its presence there is only transitory. *L. bulgaricus* is not a normal inhabitant of the intestine, nor does it survive there. *L. acidophilus*, and to a lesser extent, *L. bifidus*, are the only strains of *Lactobacillus* that are present normally in the large intestine. The strains can be implanted successfully.

LONG-TERM OUTCOME OF EARLY INVESTIGATIONS

Looking back, Metchnikoff's contributions were valuable. He did report that lactic acid bacteria made it impossible for many disease- or toxic-producing microbes to thrive and multiply. He concluded that by reducing or destroying the pathogenic microbes in the intestinal tract, many digestive as well as chronic, degenerative diseases could be eliminated. This radical conclusion was not accepted in his time, but ultimately led to a new medical approach and field of research, emphasizing natural methods to restore and maintain good health. Unfortunately, the primitive facilities at the time limited Metchnikoff's research. Later, his disciples, Tissier and Kellogg, would demonstrate that yogurt was not the sole factor in health restoration and maintenance. Additional factors, including other dietary components, were important for consideration.

Later, it was found that nearly always, some lactic acid bacteria, which are present in infancy, remain in the human colon. These friendly intestinal flora require lactose-rich foods on which to feed and multiply, and to be capable of overwhelming pathogenic microbes present. This finding strengthened Metchnikoff's hypothesis about the life-destroying and life-giving forces. Excellent forces to overwhelm the pathogenic microbes are present in yogurt and its whey.

Metchnikoff's great contribution was to stress the important linkage between diet and health. He maintained that the body has its own systems and mechanisms that help prevent both infectious and chronic diseases. By strengthening the immune system, probiotics such as yogurt and other lacto-fermented foods contribute to good health and healing. Currently, there is growing interest in probiotics (both foods and supplements). This interest has been stimulated by an ever-expanding body of research findings. Now we shall examine some of the science-based evidence justifying Metchnikoff's enthusiasm for yogurt.

CHAPTER 6

Yogurt and
the Gastrointestinal Tract

Metchnikoff's investigations with yogurt focused mainly on its benefits to the health of the gastrointestinal (GI) tract. He was prescient. Today, probiotics such as yogurt have become more important than ever in helping to keep the GI tract healthy.

GI disorders are common in the United States. According to the American College of Gastroenterology in Arlington, Virginia, more than 95 million Americans experience some type of digestive problem during any year. Common ailments include stomach upset, indigestion, reflux (heartburn), diarrhea, and constipation. More serious conditions include stomach ulcers and colon cancer. Each year, more than 10 million Americans are hospitalized due to GI disorders. The total annual care cost for these cases is estimated to exceed $40 billion. Whether the GI disorder is mild and transient, chronic, or severe and life threatening, probiotics can play beneficial roles by enhancing bowel health and functions.

PROBIOTICS FIGHT INFECTION

Probiotics can play important roles in combating two grave and growing problems mentioned earlier: foodborne infections and antibiotic resistance. Several different mechanisms may be responsible for probiotic bacteria's ability to help ward off foodborne infections. The probiotic bacteria in yogurt can

- resist enteric pathogens (pathogens within the intestine) by secretory immune substances

- alter the intestinal environment so as to make it less hospitable for pathogens to colonize

- achieve this alteration by acidifying the pH of the GI tract, as well as

33

with short-chain fatty acids and bacteriocins (antibacterial substances produced by certain strains of bacteria that are harmful to other bacterial strains within the same family)

- influence the population of gut flora in the GI tract

- adhere to the intestinal mucosa (membranes that line all the body passages that are in contact with air) and disrupt attempts by pathogens to adhere to the mucosa

- increase mucin production (secretions from the mucosa) and interfere with pathogen attachment to epithelial cells (cells that form membranes and tissues covering internal and external surfaces of the body and its organs)

- alter toxin-binding sites within the GI tract

(For a discussion of the specific probiotic bacteria that support health, see Chapter 11.)

Some infections, formerly regarded as benign and self-limiting, or readily treatable with antibiotics, have become more serious and recalcitrant. For example, *Staphylococcus aureus,* an infectious pathogen especially prevalent in hospital environments, has become resistant to methicillin, an antibiotic that formerly controlled this pathogen. Also, antibiotics kill the beneficial as well as the pathogenic organisms in the GI tract, making it vulnerable to infections.

Some potentially grave infectious diseases, or their treatments, destroy the beneficial flora in the GI tract. Probiotics can restore the flora.

For example, a diarrheal disease, associated with antibiotic therapy, is caused by *Clostridium difficile,* an opportunistic pathogen. Infection from this pathogen disrupts normal microflora in the intestine when antibiotic treatment is administered. Alternative treatment is needed. To restore normal intestinal microflora, yogurt can be helpful.

Campylobacter jejuni is thought to be the leading cause of bacterial gastroenteritis (chronic stomach inflammation). This pathogenic microbe can cause Guillain-Barré syndrome, an autoimmune disorder, which, among other effects, can lead to acute neuromuscular paralysis in a small number of people.

Some foodborne pathogens are potentially life threatening. An example is the virulent enterohemorrhagic *Escherichia coli* 0157:H7. This pathogen causes bloody diarrhea, colitis, and a range of serious health disorders.

The rotavirus is a common cause of diarrhea in young children. However, it is now recognized that rotavirus infections also occur in adults, as evidenced by outbreaks. The Centers for Disease Control (CDC) advised investigators and clinicians to check out the rotavirus as a possible cause of acute gastroenteritis in adults.

Rotavirus-induced diarrhea kills nearly a million children each year in developing countries. It occurs in developed countries, too, but far less frequently.

Yogurt and Travelers' Diarrhea

If you plan to travel, especially in developing countries, be aware of travelers' diarrhea. This term covers numerous infectious foodborne and waterborne pathogens that are pervasive. Any "shots" you have been given will not necessarily protect you from these infections.

To prepare for the trip, eat at least half a cup (4 ounces) of good quality, plain, whole-milk yogurt daily for at least two weeks before your departure. Also, plan to pack some trustworthy probiotic supplements you can take during the trip, along with handwipes and liquid handwash to use during your travel.

In addition, take the usual precautions. Observe the cleanliness of restaurants, their food preparers and servers, and their bathrooms. Avoid street-vended and marketplace foods. Limit your food choices to those that are well cooked and served piping hot. Shun raw foods. Drink only bottled water and use it for toothbrushing. Drink hot beverages and avoid cold ones. Do not believe the popular notion that alcoholic drinks offer protection against contaminated foods and beverages. They do not. Wash your hands frequently and thoroughly with hot soapy water, if available. Otherwise, use the handwipes and liquid handwash.

If you plan to travel on a cruise, ask your travel agent about which cruise lines have had good records of food and drink safety. Also, the Centers for Disease Control and Prevention (CDC), maintain records of outbreaks of foodborne and waterborne infections on specific cruise ships, as well as other food-travel health information on the CDC website: wwwn.cdc.gov/travel. This information is available to the public.

All these measures combined should lessen your risks of being infected with travelers' diarrhea. Safe and healthy journeying!

Generally, rotavirus infections are treated with vaccine. Some products had to be withdrawn from use after having caused serious intestinal blockage that killed some treated children.

Usually, individuals who become infected with rotavirus are treated with oral or intravenous salt and sugar solutions to prevent dehydration. Several different research studies, conducted during the 1980s and 1990s, suggested that probiotics might be a useful adjunct in rotavirus treatment.

Helicobacter pylori is a pathogenic microbe associated with stomach infection, chronic gastritis, peptic ulcer, and if untreated, can lead to gastric cancer. The ability of probiotic bacteria to influence *H. pylori* beneficially has been studied in animal tests. Results appeared promising.

Epidemiological and research evidence suggests that intestinal mucosal immunity diminishes with age. Thus, the elderly are especially vulnerable to infectious diseases, including those in the GI tract.

PROBIOTICS HELP PREVENT CONSTIPATION AND OTHER GI PROBLEMS

Constipation, dubbed the "national complaint" in the United Kingdom, is also common in the United States. It warrants discussion. Constipation is another condition experienced in the GI tract. Sometimes constipation is induced by antibiotics or by other medications that destroy the beneficial flora in the GI tract. The use of orally (or even rectally) administered yogurt has been found useful to restore the flora and relieve the constipation.

Constipation may be chronic. Note the number of over-the-counter laxatives on the shelves in drug stores and supermarkets, and the number of advertisements for commercial products pitched to produce "regularity." Also, harsh measures with home remedies include enemas, and herbal mixes with senna leaves. One remedy, submitted to the journal *Gut*, consisted of dandelion leaves boiled with a lump of coal, as a remedy for severe constipation!

Draconian measures are unnecessary to relieve constipation. Many cases result from faulty dietary choices involving an inadequate intake of fruits, vegetables, whole grains, and water. These foods provide dietary fiber, and the water, lubrication. Too little exercise may be an additional factor. Using commercial psyllium-containing products, such as Metamucil, intended to provide dietary fiber is unnecessary. Also, some people are allergic to psyllium. The simple solution is to increase the intake of

Yogurt as a Bactericide

Experimental inoculation of yogurt with some of the world's most dreaded infectious disease organisms has provided dramatic proof of yogurt as a potent bactericide. Yogurt has demonstrated its ability to fight infections such as typhus, anthrax, dysentery, tuberculosis, meningitis, diptheria, pneumonia, and others. These are some of the findings with yogurt inoculations:

- *Salmonella typhi* died within thirty to forty-eight hours.

- *Escherichia coli* were unable to develop.

- *Salmonella paratyphi* and *Corynebacterium diphtheriae* lost their pathogenicity.

- *Neisseria meningitides* and *Vibrio comma* lost their virulence.

- Pathogenic or saprophytic bacteria (bacteria that grow on, and derive their nourishment from decaying or dead organic matter) seldom were found after being inoculated with yogurt containing from 1.65 to 2 percent lactic acid.

- *E. coli, Streptococcus* and *Staphylococcus* were killed in dahi, a fermented yogurt-type milk consumed in India. The dahi did not kill but inhibited *S. typhi.*

- *V. comma,* added to yogurt, died within the first five minutes; *S. typhi,* within one hour, and *Shigella,* within two hours. The acidity of the yogurt was critical. When the pH of the yogurt was raised by the addition of a neutralizing (alkaline) agent, the pathogens were able to survive.

- Even month-old yogurt was found to have bactericidal effects on pathogenic microbes that are not controlled by commonly used therapeutic antibiotics. (However, it is desirable to eat freshly cultured yogurt.)

- The whey from yogurt made with cow's milk displayed a wide spectrum of bactericidal properties. Pathogenic bacteria such as *S. typhi, S. paratyphi, Shigella paradysenteriae, Brucella abortus* (the pathogen responsible for brucellosis in cows), *V. comma,* and *Bacillus subtilis* were all killed within one hour; *Shigella dysenteriae, Pseudomonas vulgaris,* and *Salmonella pullorum* within two hours; *E. coli* and *Klebsiella pneumoniae,* within five hours; and *C. diphtheriae* within twenty-four hours.

fibrous foods. Eat the orange rather than drink orange juice; eat the apple rather than drink apple juice; and eat the tomato rather than drink tomato juice. In partitioning food, most or all of the fiber is removed from the juice.

Yogurt is also useful to alleviate constipation. As early as 1955, Drs. Francis Ferrer and Linn J. Boyd reported that the use of yogurt (in a prune whip) had beneficial effects on constipation. Ferrer and Boyd found that the addition of prunes to plain yogurt did not affect the yogurt's bacterial flora or its physiological effect. They fed the yogurt-prune mixture to 194 hospitalized, chronically ill, elderly patients who suffered from constipation. A few of the patients refused to take the mixture. Of those who did, 187 patients (95.8 percent) required no laxative during the time they ate the yogurt-prune mixture. Only seven (4.2 percent) of the patients had to resort to a laxative. In addition to the beneficial relief of constipation, there were other rewards. The patients' skin tone improved. Seborrheic dermatitis (a coating of oil, crust, or scale on the skin) decreased. There were decreases in chronic ileus (an intestinal obstruction that can cause constipation, colic, and vomiting), as well as diabetic ulcers.

Other GI health problems that respond favorably to probiotics include

- patients with chronic kidney and liver diseases, who have pathogenic overgrowth in the small bowel of the intestinal tract with toxic amines in the bloodstream

- inflammatory bowel disease (IBD), including Crohn's disease and ulcerative colitis

- irritable bowel syndrome (IBS), also called spastic colon or mucous colitis

- pseudomenbranous colitis, induced by *Clostridium difficile*

In addition, rat studies showed some beneficial effects of probiotics with the problem of intestinal permeability to antigens. (Intestinal permeability allows substances that the body perceives as foreign to enter the bloodstream, where they induce allergic reactions. Antigens are substances foreign to the body. To combat them, the immune system produces antibodies.) Other rat studies demonstrated that probiotics could neutralize cholera toxins.

Probiotics can play a role in fostering good health and functioning in the GI tract, which is linked to proper functioning of the immune system. Next, this connection is discussed.

CHAPTER 7

Yogurt and the Immune System

The body's immune system has many vital functions. It responds to foreign substances that enter the body, including foods, toxins, pathogens, foreign blood cells from transfusions, and cells of foreign organs from transplantations, by producing combative antibodies.

A strong immune system, functioning in a healthy body, responds to antigens by launching protective reactions. As examples, the immune system launches an attack on food allergens in the gastrointestinal (GI) tract. Or, the immune system initiates an assault on pathogenic microbes that attempt to colonize in the GI tract.

A poorly functioning immune system, in a weakened body, lacks the vigor to protect the body from allergic and inflammatory reactions that, over time, can lead to serious health problems. The immune system can be compromised in individuals with certain health conditions, who are given immune-suppression medication. Disease states impair the functioning of the immune system. Also, as the body ages, the immune system functions less efficiently.

The GI tract—from mouth to anus—is the body's largest area of mucosal surface in contact with antigens (such as foods, toxins, and pathogens). The lymph tissue lining the gut transforms the GI tract into the largest immune organ in the human body. Approximately 80 percent of all immunoglobulin-producing cells in the body are produced in the GI tract.

PROBIOTICS STIMULATE IMMUNE FUNCTION

Immunoglobulins are proteins with antibody activity that are found in serum and other body fluids and tissues. Immunoglobulins are divided into classes, based on their structure and antigenic properties. IgA is the main antibody in the membrane of both the GI tract and the respiratory

Bacteria and the Immune System

"Most people are surprised to hear that a normal human being hosts a mass of bacteria equivalent to about 1.2 kilograms: the bulk are in the gut lumen, and the remaining [bacteria] mainly dispersed among the skin, the rhino-oral-pharyngeal cavities, and the genital mucosae. Their weight almost equals that of the liver . . . they are smaller than our cells, and their total number . . . exceeds that of our own cells. It is also most incredible that over 400 species . . . are well adapted to particular environments such as gingival crevices, and the intestinal and vaginal niches, enjoying the wealth of nutrients and the constancy of temperature . . . Bacteria came before us and most likely will remain for some time after our extinction. Meanwhile, they thrive on us and send us continuous signals with which the immune system keeps them at bay . . ."

—Velio Bocci, Institute of General Physiology and Nutritional Sciences, University of Siena, Italy, 1992

tract. ("Ig" stands for immunoglobulin.) Due to immunoglobulins, the digestive tract can elicit a variety of immunologic responses from many different local cells.

Through this mechanism, researchers suggest that probiotic bacteria, as biologic response modifiers, can influence immune responses. Studies suggest that probiotic bacteria are able to enhance non-specific as well as specific immune responses, in different ways. They can

- mediate immune activity by means of fermented products and from viable probiotic cells, without provoking a harmful inflammatory response

- activate macrophages (large cells in the walls of blood vessels and in loose connective tissues, usually immobile but mobilized by inflammation)

- increase levels of cytokines (substances responsible for cell division and tissue differentiation, as well as for stimulating both humoral and cellular immune responses)

- increase the activity of natural killer cells

- increase the level of immunoglobulins, especially IgA

Probiotics such as yogurt enhance immune functioning. As mentioned earlier, probiotics help protect against viral and bacterial pathogens. Also, probiotics help inhibit tumor formation. Researchers have been able to measure these effects.

Non-specific immune responses are a host's first line of defense. Natural killer cells and phagocytes (substances that can envelop and destroy harmful bacteria and other foreign substances) residing in the peripheral blood and tissues are the major cellular effectors of non-specific immunity.

Natural killer cells effectively combat viruses; phagocyte cells protect against microbial infections. Both produce a variety of compounds that can destroy invasive materials.

There are two specific immune responses: humoral and cell-mediated. In the humoral immune response, B-lymphocytes (products of lymph tissue that participate in immune response) synthesize specific immunoglobulin molecules (antibodies) that are excreted from the cell and bind to the invading substance. In the cellular immune response, T-lymphocytes, having immunoglobulin-like molecules on their surfaces, recognize and kill foreign as well as aberrant cells (cells that deviate from normal ones).

Certain probiotic strains of bacteria in fermented foods enhance non-specific immunity by proliferating phagocytes and lymphocytes. This development demonstrates that probiotics stimulate cellular immune responses.

PROBIOTCS SUPPORT IMMUNE RESPONSE

In 1991, George Halpern and his colleagues at the University of California School of Medicine at Davis conducted the first large-scale study of yogurt's effects on the human immune system of sixty-eight individuals, twenty to forty years of age. One-third consumed yogurt with live active cultures; one-third, yogurt that had been heated to deactivate the inoculated bacteria (a practice of some yogurt manufacturers); and one-third (the control), consumed no yogurt. After four months, the group consuming the yogurt with the live active cultures had increased their levels of interferon *fivefold* over the other groups. Interferon is a class of small proteins released by cells that have been invaded by a virus. They are the immune system's first line of defense against viral infections. The researchers admitted that two cups of yogurt as part of the daily diet— the amount used in the study—might be unrealistically high for many people. But Halpern suggested that even one cup of yogurt daily would be sufficient to help fight infections (*Internatl J Immunol*, Mar 1991).

Several years later, in another study, twenty-eight volunteers were given several glasses of milk daily that had been inoculated either with *Lactobacillus acidophilus* or *Bifidobacterium bifidum*. After three weeks, the ability of the participants to manufacture phagocytes *nearly doubled*. Six weeks after the participants stopped drinking the treated milk, their ability to increase the production of phagocytes remained substantially above normal, but had decreased from the former high level achieved during the study (*Am J Clin Nutr*, 1997).

In one study, consumption of *Bacillus lactis* was associated with an increase in the total proportion of T-lymphocytes to natural killer cells. Another study strengthened this finding. Healthy middle-aged and elderly men and women experienced significant enhancement of phagocytes and natural killer-cell activity against tumors after eating *B. lactis* twice daily. The researchers suggested that much of the enhanced immunity might be related to the secretion of potent immunity cytokines known as interleukins. The interleukins stimulate natural killer-cell activity and interferon production. The interferon induces in non-infected cells the formation of an antiviral protein that inhibits viral proliferation.

Chronic tobacco smoking reduces the body's ability to produce natural killer cells. In 2005, ninety-nine habitual cigarette-smoking Japanese men, twenty-four to sixty years of age, with poor to moderately good health practices in addition to their smoking habit, volunteered to participate in a study. They were given a fermented milk product containing *Lactobacillus casei*. The results showed that the number of cigarettes smoked daily correlated inversely with natural killer-cell activity: the more cigarettes smoked, the less killer-cell activity. The researchers suggested that probiotics, by enhancing the immune system, might be an effective means to restore killer-cell activity lost through habitual smoking.

PROBIOTICS PROTECT A WEAKENED IMMUNE SYSTEM

Probiotics play a vital role in the intestinal mucosal barrier, by modulating the intestinal immune response, and inhibiting adhesion of pathogenic microbes to the epithelial wall of the intestine. The intestinal epithelium plays an important role in innate immunity. When stimulated by cytokines, the intestinal epithelia release pro-inflammatory cytokines. However, in gastrointestinal diseases such as irritable bowel disease (IBD) and acute gastroenteritis, the activated cytokines produce excessive inflammatory products that adversely affect the immunological capacity of the epithelium cells. In such circumstances, probiotics with *Bifidobacterium* and *Lactobacillus* help quench the pro-inflammatory response by retarding the secretion of pro-inflammatory cytokines. This ability of probiotics to inhibit a potentially dysfunctioning immune system has wide application. It could benefit individuals with autoimmune diseases and other disorders that are accompanied by inflammation, such as rheumatoid arthritis and IBD. Ingestion of specific probiotics has immunomodulatory effects on humoral and cell-mediated immunity.

Now that the links between the immune system, the GI tract, and probiotics have been established, let's examine some of the specific responses—food allergies, intolerances, sensitivities, and other health problems—that are related to these linkages.

CHAPTER 8

Yogurt and Food Allergy, Intolerance, and Sensitivity

The terms food allergy, food intolerance, and food sensitivity are frequently, but wrongly, used interchangeably to refer to adverse reactions induced by certain foods. They are distinctly different disorders.

Food allergy is a complex immune response by an antibody to an antigen. Antibodies can be in circulating blood throughout the body, attached to cells in various parts of the body, and on various body surfaces. Some common symptoms include mucous production, runny nose, and bronchial swelling. Symptoms may be acute or delayed.

Food intolerance is an adverse reaction that can result from various mechanisms, including enzyme deficiencies and metabolic disease, among others. An individual with food intolerance experiences digestive discomfort after eating certain foods. For example, someone with lactose intolerance may react to dairy products due to a deficiency of the enzyme, lactase; or someone with gluten intolerance may react to gluten-containing grains such as wheat and rye.

Food sensitivity leads to a reaction induced regularly by exposure to a food (or related ones) and a specific antibody is detectable. For example, buckwheat, rhubarb, and garden sorrel are all in the same plant family. If an individual is sensitive to buckwheat, then it would be prudent to avoid rhubarb and garden sorrel, as well as buckwheat.

As one might surmise, food allergies, food intolerances, and food sensitivities are related to the gastrointestinal (GI) tract. The good news is that yogurt and other cultured dairy foods can play a beneficial role with these conditions.

PROBIOTIC'S ANTI-ALLERGY EFFECTS

Food allergies are increasing in the United States. The Food and Drug

Administration (FDA) estimates that about 5 percent of infants and young children, and 2 percent of adults, have food allergies. The eight major allergenic foods in the American food supply are peanuts, soybeans, wheat, milk, eggs, finfish, crustacean shellfish, and tree nuts. However, dozens of other foods can be allergenic for some people. Any food, despite its wholesomeness, can be allergenic.

The eight major allergenic foods happen to be ones that are used extensively, and repeatedly, in the typical American diet. As examples, the rise in peanut allergy correlates with the rise in the all-too-common practice of feeding peanut butter and jelly sandwiches to children, day after day. Or, the proliferation of soybean, in many guises, in processed foods, has made this formerly benign food rise to become a major allergen.

Typically, allergens induce mucosal inflammation in the GI tract. They

How to Minimize Allergic Reactions

Eat a wide variety of basic foods, and avoid, insofar as possible, highly processed ones. By eating a wide variety, you break the undesirable feature of eating specific foods constantly. Highly processed foods contain a few components such as corn, soybean, or wheat, in many guises. Read the labels on packaged cereals. The ingredients are basically similar, but with different shapes or flavorings. The variety is illusionary. Highly processed foods narrow the food base, and do not offer real variety.

Rotate your food. This is a wise practice, even for those who do not have food allergies. By not eating the same food day after day after day, you minimize the possibility of a buildup of allergic reactions. For example, instead of eating oatmeal for breakfast daily, rotate it with other wholegrains such as brown rice, quinoa, barley, amaranth, and so forth.

Take note of what your GI tract is telling you. After eating a specific food, does your digestive system produce reflux, discomfort, cramps, flatus, diarrhea, or other signs of intestinal distress? Is the gas merely from having eaten onions or beans, or from a food that does not usually produce gas? To detect an allergic reaction from a specific food, keep a food diary. You may be able to pinpoint the food that is causing the distress. Eliminate it for a while, then challenge yourself by eating it. If the distress returns, your suspicion is confirmed. If your reaction is severe, avoid the can alter gut motility, and frequently, malabsorption of nutrients, diarrhea, and abdominal pain ensue. Probiotics can alter the balance of bacteria in the gut, and boost the immune system.

Cow's milk allergy is experienced by some infants and young children. The intact proteins in the milk stimulate the secretion of pro-inflammatory cytokines. Specific strains of lactic acid bacteria promote the integrity of the gut mucosal barrier, and protect these children from sensitization. *Lactobacillus rhamnosus*, especially, dampens hypersensitive reactions and intestinal inflammation in food-sensitive individuals. These benefits are achieved mainly by improving the antigen-specific immune responses, and in modulating the antigen absorption into the mucosal membrane.

A breakdown of the mucosal barrier function allows the GI tract to be

---

food; if mild, eat it infrequently, and in small amounts. If the reaction still occurs, avoid the food.

In attempting to learn which food is causing the problem, eat only a few foods at the same time. Select those that you know agree with you, and one that you suspect does not.

Even better, in sorting out the problem, eat only one food that you suspect is causing the problem. This procedure was formulated in "the pulse test" devised by an eminent allergist, Arthur F. Coca, M.D. This diagnostic test is simple and requires no special equipment other than a watch with a second hand. It is best to conduct the test when you are home for some days. In a sitting position, take your pulse fourteen times during the day: once when you rise and once when you retire; once before each of three meals; and at half-hour intervals three times after each of the three meals. Record each pulse along with the single food eaten. The pulse rates on arising, retiring, and before meals serve as a base line. After eating the single food, if your pulse rate goes up dramatically, consider that this rise has been caused by an allergic reaction to the food.

Become acquainted with food plant families. For example, the nightshade family includes eggplant, potato, tomato, peppers of all kinds, ground cherry, as well as tobacco. If you have reactions to one food in the family, avoid other foods in the same family as well.

challenged by allergens. Probiotic bacteria can improve the mucosal barrier function, and thus, lessen allergic reactions.

A 1993 study by C. G. Trapp and colleagues divided college-aged and elderly individuals into three groups. For twelve months, the first group ate yogurt that contained live and active bacteria; the second, pasteurized yogurt; and the third, no yogurt. There was a significant decrease in allergic symptoms in the first group compared to the others. (Unfortunately, some yogurt producers pasteurize their products after the yogurt is produced, in order to extend the shelflife. This practice deactivates the useful bacteria and defeats the purpose of eating yogurt for its special benefits bestowed by live active bacteria.)

A 1996 study by L. Pelto and associates measured the phagocytes in eight adults who were hypersensitive to milk, but were not lactose intolerant. The participants could tolerate milk containing *Lactobacillus* GG, but not regular milk. This strain of bacterium may suppress a milk-induced-immune inflammatory response.

Studies in Finland supported these claims. In 1993, Erika Isolauri and her colleagues from the Department of Pediatrics at the Medical School of the University of Tempere, showed that probiotics can be helpful in managing food allergies. They found that the strain of *L.* GG promoted local antigen-specific immune responses, especially IgA. Also, they found that it prevented gut permeability and control of antigen absorption. Four years later, Dr. Isolauri and her colleague, Hell Majamaa, demonstrated that patients with food allergies were helped by probiotics. Cow's milk, inoculated with *L.* GG, alleviated intestinal inflammation.

PROBIOTICS IMPROVE FOOD INTOLERANCE

A noteworthy application of yogurt and other cultured dairy foods is in lactose intolerance. Individuals with this condition have difficulty digesting regular milk, but usually can tolerate fermented milk.

Lactose intolerance (less commonly termed lactose malabsorption or lactose maldigestion) is an inability to digest milk because of a deficiency of lactase (an enzyme) needed to digest lactose (the milk sugar). It is estimated that about 30 million Americans are lactose intolerant. Worldwide, estimates run as high as 90 percent. Indeed, it might be regarded that those who are lactose tolerant, in the minority, have an aberrant condition!

Most people have large amounts of lactase at birth, except for a rare number of newborns who lack lactase. In cultures where dairy foods continue to be consumed after weaning, during childhood and adulthood, the people continue to produce lactase and consume dairy foods. These groups are notably from northern and western Europe, and the Masai in Africa. In cultures where dairy foods are not consumed after weaning, the lactase production declines. These groups are Africans, Asians, Native Americans, and Afro-Americans, among others.

Tolerance for lactose varies widely. Some individuals can tolerate very little or no milk; others can tolerate somewhat more. Usually, tolerance is better if the milk is consumed along with food during a meal, rather than by itself between meals. The accompanying food reduces the concentration of lactose by slowing the stomach's emptying time. Fat-containing food is helpful. For example, chocolate-flavored milk

Confirming Lactose Intolerance

If you suspect that you are lactose intolerant, simple procedures can offer evidence. Avoid all dairy products and products that contain dairy constituents. Read carefully the ingredient listings on labels. Even so-called non-dairy creamers may contain milk fractions.

After avoiding all dairy foods for a week or two, note whether you no longer have signs of gastrointestinal distress. If so, challenge yourself by consuming some dairy foods, and observe whether or not the gastrointestinal distress returns. If it does, avoid fresh milk, but switch to a small amount of cultured milk products such as yogurt, buttermilk, acidophilus, kefir, and aged cheeses. Note whether or not you can tolerate them. If you can tolerate them, you have evidence of lactose intolerance. If you cannot tolerate them, suspect milk allergy. With true milk allergy, it is necessary to exclude totally all dairy foods, and the exclusion should be lifetime.

If you wish to have a medical confirmation of suspected lactose intolerance, there are two noninvasive procedures used in a medical setting such as a hospital. One diagnostic test is an oral lactose intolerance test based on routine laboratory procedure. The other is a breath hydrogen test, which is regarded as more reliable. This test is useful for evaluating lactose digestion.

may be tolerated better than plain milk, due to the fat in the chocolate. Skim milk and reduced-fat milk are poorly tolerated because of the loss or reduction of fat. Also, such products have what consumers describe as a "skinny" taste. To the food processor, this is known as an organoleptic lack of good "mouthfeel." To compensate, non-fat milk powder is added to skim milk and reduced-fat milk to achieve more "body." The non-fat milk powder contains lactose. Addition of the powder increases the total amount of lactose in these products, and makes it even harder for lactose intolerant individuals to digest them.

In the culturing process, much of the lactose is hydrolyzed by the bacterial cultures used in the fermentation process. Hence, lactase is not needed to digest such products. Aged cheeses such as cheddar and Swiss may be tolerated, whereas fresh cheeses such as cottage cheese and farmer cheese that still contain lactose may not be well tolerated. Skim-milk cheeses are poorly tolerated for the same reason that skim milk and reduced-fat milks are not tolerated. Yogurt, kefir, and other fermented dairy products are tolerated, unless the processor decides to boost the product with additional non-fat milk powder.

Whole-milk yogurt is tolerated better than regular fluid milk. Yogurt's bacteria survive gastric digestion and are active in the GI tract. Hence, the bacteria can substitute for the individual's own lactase that might be low or lacking.

Cultured buttermilk does not change lactose digestion significantly, because only a small amount of lactose is metabolized by its bacteria. For the same reason, the action of sweet acidophilus milk is equivalent to that of regular fluid milk. It does not alleviate the distressful symptoms for a lactose-intolerant individual.

Commercial products are available with food-grade lactases (beta-galactosidase enzyme preparations from microbial organisms). They are used to produce lactose-hydrolyzed milk and other reduced-lactose products. They can be substituted for regular fluid milk. They contain from 40 to 90 percent less lactose than regular milk. Some dairies make such products available.

Another approach to make regular fluid milk better tolerated is to use commercially available lactose-reducing products. One is Lactaid, which is added to milk at home. To be fully effective, such products require a twenty-four-hour incubation period.

PROBIOTICS ALLEVIATE ALLERGY-RELATED HEALTH PROBLEMS

Respiratory ailments, gastrointestinal problems, eczema, and other seemingly unrelated conditions can be manifestations of allergy. They can also be improved with probiotics.

Respiratory and GI Infections

Respiratory and gastrointestinal problems can be related to allergies. Infants and young children who attend childcare centers have a higher incidence of gastroenteritis and respiratory illnesses than children who do not attend. One study was conducted in Israel over twenty-one months by Zvi Weizman and associates. They studied infants, aged four to ten months in fourteen different childcare centers. The children were given either *Lactobacillus reuteri* or *Bifidobacteria lactis*. The number of episodes and total number of days that the children experienced respiratory illness, diarrhea, or fever were all recorded. The results showed that the *L. reuteri*-treated group had a better overall effect on all parameters than *B. lactis*.

Similar studies were conducted in Finland by Katja Hatakka and associates at the Foundation for Nutrition Research in Helsinki. The researchers attempted to learn whether long-term consumption of a probiotic-fortified milk could reduce gastrointestinal and respiratory infections in children in fifteen different daycare centers. The beneficial bacterium *L.* GG was given to 571 healthy children, aged one to six years, and 289 healthy children of similar ages in the control group. The results of the study showed that *L.* GG can reduce both respiratory and gastrointestinal infections and their severity in children in daycare centers.

Allergic rhinopathy, a disease of the nasal mucous membrane, is another disorder helped by yogurt. In a study by C. Aldinucci and colleagues, adults who had allergic rhinopathy, aged nineteen to forty-four years, were given either 450 grams of yogurt or low-fat milk daily for four months. There were no other dietary changes. At the end of the four months, the participants who had consumed the yogurt showed significant improvement; those on the low-fat milk consumption showed no improvement.

The nose can harbor potentially pathogenic bacteria. In a study con-

ducted by U. Glück and J. O. Gebbers, 209 volunteers were given a probiotic-supplemented milk drink that was cultured with L. GG, *Bifidobacterium* sp. 3420 (one specie), *L. acidophilus*, and *Streptococcus thermophilus*, or
they were given standard yogurt, cultured with the conventional lactic
acid bacteria *S. thermophilus* and *Lactobacillus delbrueckii* subsp. (subspecies) *bulgaricus*. The volunteers consumed the yogurt daily for three
weeks. Then, the nasal flora were examined. In the group that had consumed the probiotic-supplemented milk drink, the number of individuals
who had potentially pathogenic bacteria in the nasal cavity decreased
significantly. In the group that had consumed the standard yogurt, potentially pathogenic bacteria were found in the nasal cavity throughout the
study period. The pathogenic bacteria identified included *Staphyloccocus
aureus, Streptococcus pneumonia*, beta-hemolytic *Streptococci*, and *Haemophilus
influenzae*. The study results suggested a link between lymph tissue in the
gut and the upper respiratory tract.

Improves Allergy-Related Eczema

Infants with eczema (atopic dermatitis)—another manifestation of allergy
—who received a formula supplemented with L. GG showed significant
improvement in the severity of this skin ailment, compared to infants
who did not receive this probiotic.

Drs. Majamaa and Isolauri, whose investigations with allergies were
discussed earlier, also studied the use of probiotics with cases of eczema
in infants. They noted earlier misunderstandings about the role of food
allergy in atopic dermatitis. Their own studies suggested that dietary antigens contributed to the worsening of eczema in some infants. An elimina-
tion diet helped and was able to reverse some of the disturbances in
immune responses to the dietary antigens. Majamaa and Isolauri demonstrated, for the first time, the ability of probiotic treatment to eliminate
dietary antigens and restore intestinal barrier function. In their study, the
strain of the probiotic chosen was L. GG, which has been shown to survive passage through the intestinal tract and to colonize, transiently, in
the gut. The researchers noted significant clinical improvement, both in
limiting the extent and the intensity of eczema in the treated infants.

In a Danish study, a team led by Vibeke Rosenfeldt gave forty-three
children with atopic dermatitis, aged one to thirteen years, a *Lactobacillus*
supplement for six weeks, followed by a placebo for six weeks. During
the time of the *Lactobacillus* treatment, 56 percent of the children had sig-

nificantly fewer symptoms of eczema. The children had a 15 percent reduction of symptoms when they consumed the placebo.

The same group of researchers conducted another study. They found that the use of *Lactobacillus* supplements reduced gut permeability and GI distress. Gut permeability allows undigested proteins to enter the bloodstream, where they induce allergic reactions such as eczema and asthma.

Although probiotics such as yogurt have demonstrated their beneficial effects with food allergies, food intolerances, food sensitivities, and related problems of respiratory ailments, there are still more beneficial effects with various organs, systems, and diseases. Next, let's look at yogurt's beneficial effects on the genitourinary tract.

CHAPTER 9

Yogurt and
the Genitourinary Tract

As already noted, the development of infections in the urinary/vaginal tract, as well as in the gastrointestinal tract, may occur when the normal microflora are disrupted by antibiotics, medications, or medical procedures. Multiple mechanisms exist for actions by biotherapeutic agents such as probiotics to stop pathogenic proliferation until normal microflora can be reestablished. The biotherapeutic agents produce antimicrobial substances. For example, *Lactobacillus casei* GG produces a very small non-pathogenic bacterium called a microcin that inhibits a broad spectrum of pathogens.

For centuries, crude mixtures of fermented milk products have been used to treat yeast infections known as *Candida albicans* or candidal vaginitis, a recurrent yeast infection in the vaginal tract. With the advent of modern medicine and use of antibiotics, the old tradition waned. But, it was never totally eclipsed. Yogurt consumption continues to be a household remedy. Yogurt and *Lactobacillus acidophilus*-containing milk even are used in solutions for vaginal douches to treat this condition. The medical establishment, by and large, dismissed these practices as worthless.

Among many infections that can occur in the genitourinary tract, recurrent candidal vaginitis is only one, but a very common one among American women. Other infections include gonorrhea, *Trichomonas*, and the human immune deficiency virus (HIV).

An increased incidence of candidal vaginitis is noted in women who are pregnant, diabetic, or treated with antibiotics or corticosteroids. However, women can experience chronic yeast infections from other causes, including poor dietary habits. For example, a high intake of sugar exacerbates the yeast problem because yeasts feed on sugars.

Current prophylactic therapies admittedly are inadequate. Antibiotic treatment does not prevent recurrence, and can have negative side effects. Can yogurt, long used in folk remedy, eliminate candidal vaginitis, as well as prevent its recurrence? With the alarming problems of antibiotic resistance, and the side effects from antibiotic treatments, the medical establishment has taken a fresh look at yogurt and other cultured milk products as potential treatments for vaginal yeast infections and other genitourinary infections.

PROBIOTICS SUPPORT GENITOURINARY HEALTH

In the healthy vagina, lactobacilli are the predominant microorganisms. They contribute to vaginal health by producing lactic acid, and by maintaining a relatively acidic environment.

Vaginal yeast infection is associated with a lack of lactobacilli. Some lactobacilli produce hydrogen peroxide, a powerful bactericide that can be toxic to organisms that produce little or no enzymes and are hydrogen peroxide scavengers.

In laboratory experiments, additional metabolic products of lactobacilli have been shown to inhibit pathogens. Competition for nutrients may be another mechanism for biotherapeutic agents, as well as competition for bacterial adhesion sites in the vagina and intestinal tract. Also, biotherapeutic agents may modify toxin receptors by means of enzymes. Different mechanisms may be involved, depending on the specific pathogen. The body's response to biotherapeutic agents may depend on the efficient functioning of the body's immune system.

In a study led by David A. Eschenbach, *Lactobacillus* species were found in the vagina of 96 percent of healthy women, but in only 6 percent of women with vaginal yeast infections.

Other investigators identified acidophyllin as the antibacterial component of *L. acidophilus.* Acidophyllin reduced by half the growth of numerous types of bacteria that thrive in cultures that are free of lactic acid. Ten of these bacterial types are common pathogens. Identifications were made by Khem M. Shahani and his colleagues, and reported in *Cultured Dairy Products Journal* in 1977.

Probiotics Restore Healthy Flora and Reduce Vaginal Infections

Can vaginal implantation of *L. acidophilus* inhibit recurrent *C. albicans* in women? This question was addressed in 1980 by E. B. Collins and Pamela Hardt, from the Department of Food Science and Technology, at the University of California at Davis. They chose thirty women with recurrent *C. albicans* who had been treated previously for the infection with nystatin, an antibiotic commonly used to treat vaginal infections. The researchers divided the women into two groups. The first group received a vaginal implantation of nonfermented milk inoculated with *L. acidophilus;* the second group, with regular yogurt; and the third group, with low-fat milk. After three months, there were fewer recurrences of the infection in the first and second groups. The low-fat milk given to the third group failed to prevent recurrences of the infection.

A case study that dramatized the efficacy of a single suppository with a specific strain of *Lactobacillus* was reported by Gregor Reid and his associates in 1994. A thirty-three-year-old woman had a four-year history of recurrent vaginal infections, some of which cultured positive for *C. albicans.* Concurrently, she suffered with recurrent bladder infections. A vaginal swab was taken, and it showed no lactobacilli present. The predominant infectious organism present was *Enterococcus faecalis.* A single intravaginal suppository containing *Lactobacillus casei* var. *rhamnosus GR-1* was inserted into the woman's vagina. Follow-up swabbings were taken after two, three, and seven weeks. The cultures revealed the continued presence of the identical strain of *Lactobacillus* that had been implanted originally by the single suppository. Two days after the suppository insertion, the patient had become symptom free, and remained free of both vaginal and bladder infections during the entire length of the seven-week study. During the next six months the patient received two additional suppository insertions, and at the time of the reporting of the case study, she had remained free of symptoms.

Good results were reported in Germany with direct implantation of *Lactobacillus* cultures to treat vaginal infections. G. Karkut treated ninety-four women intravaginally with a *L. acidophilus* preparation. The pathogens decreased, and at the same time, the vaginal acidity was restored to a normal level. This change permitted the *Lactobacillus* flora to colonize. About 80 percent of the women showed either a complete restoration of a normal vaginal environment, or a marked improvement of symptoms.

Live *L. Acidophilus* Bacteria Critical to Success

A study published in 1992 was hailed as the first controlled trial to demonstrate the benefits of *L. acidophilus*-containing yogurt against recurrent *C. albicans.* Eileen Hilton, a gynecologist, led a team at Long Island

Jewish Medical Center in New Hyde Park, New York, to study women with chronic vaginal yeast infection. The study began with thirty-three women, but dwindled to only thirteen women by the end of the study. (The reason for this decrease will be discussed shortly.)

The women were divided into two groups. The first group ate a cupful of plain yogurt containing live *L. acidophilus* daily for six months; the second group (the control) ate none. After six months, the women who had consumed the yogurt had only one-third as many infectious episodes as those who had not. In fact, the treated women felt so much improved that they refused to switch over as a control group, a protocol that had been designed in the study. The researchers concluded that plain yogurt containing live *L. acidophilus* was a beneficial prophylactic for candidal vaginitis.

In view of the number of participants, this study was modest. The declining number from thirty-three to thirteen individuals is instructive. In attempting to make certain that the women were confirmed cases of candidal vaginitis, the researchers made a startling discovery. More than one-fourth of the women originally considered for the study had been misdiagnosed by their own physicians. They were not infected by candidal vaginitis, but had other vaginal conditions, including gonorrhea, *Trichomonas*, and herpes virus. According to the researchers, none of these infections would be expected to respond favorably to *L. acidophilus* treatment. The implications are important. Yogurt's potential benefits as a prophylactic might appear to be less effective for candidal vaginitis than it actually is, because studies might be skewed by the inclusion of women with non-yeast vaginal infections. Results of yogurt's true benefit would be underestimated. Also, the distorted results might make skeptical gynecologists even more skeptical about yogurt's effectiveness, and make them even more reluctant to use it as a treatment for patients.

In addition to these hurdles, not all yogurt producers add *L. acidophilus*. It is not a bacterium required to culture the milk. The essential ones for culturing are *L. bulgaricus* and *Streptococcus thermophilus*. Yogurt producers may choose to add *L. acidophilus* because its perceived benefits can increase sales.

Hilton cautioned, "Those interested in using dairy products to recolonize their gastrointestinal tracts should be wary of claims of dairy manufacturers. When various brands of yogurt were tested, some did not contain the advertised lactobacilli." This finding may be an additional factor in failed cases with candidal vaginitis, and would only strengthen the doubt of the skeptics.

Commercial yogurts are not standardized. In the Hilton study, the researchers chose Columbo plain yogurt because they found that it contained a high content of supplemental *L. acidophilus*. Unfortunately, by 1992, the year of publication of Hilton's study, the Columbo plain yogurt no longer contained this beneficial microorganism, according to Herbert Keating, III, M.D., associate chairman of the Department of Medicine at the Medical Center of Delaware in Wilmington.

According to the Hilton team, *L. acidophilus* is more resistant to digestive acids than other gut bacteria. The team found higher levels of *L. acidophilus* in the rectums and vaginas of the women during the study, and attributed this finding to yogurt's ability to move its bacteria from the rectal area into the vaginal area. As Hilton reported, "It appears that the gastrointestinal strain of *L. acidophilus* colonized the vaginal tract of our patients."

Other researchers demonstrated the importance of having live *L. acidophilus* in the yogurt in order to benefit women with candidal vaginitis. In 1996, E. Shalev and associates gave twenty-three women yogurt with live *L. acidophilus*, and twenty-three women yogurt that had been pasteurized after being cultured. The women in the first group experienced more than a 50 percent reduction in recurrent infections; the second group experienced only a slight reduction.

A study of HIV-positive women who were prone to vaginal infections was reported by A. Williams in 2000. In a double-blind study, the women

Recognition Is Slow, but Coming

"There is now evidence that administration of selected microorganisms is beneficial in the prevention and treatment of certain intestinal [infectious] and, possibly, treatment of vaginal infections. In an effort to decrease the reliance on antimicrobials [antibiotics], the time has come to carefully explore the therapeutic applications of biotherapeutic agents."

—Gary W. Elmer, Ph.D., Department of Medicinal Chemistry, School of Pharmacy, University of Washington, Seattle, printed in the *Journal of the American Medical Association*, March 20, 1996 were divided into three groups. The first group was given a weekly vaginal insertion of a gelatin capsule containing *L. acidophilus*. The second group was given 100 milligrams (mg) daily of clotrimazole, a drug commonly used for vaginal infections. The third group (the control) was given a placebo. Over a period of about twenty-one months, the group given *L. acidophilus* experienced beneficial results that were nearly as good as those who had been given the drug; they also had only half the risk of the control group in experiencing additional episodes of candidal infection.

Other *Lactobacillus* Strains Prove Valuable

Although much of the research with beneficial bacteria for control of candidal vaginitis has been focused on *L. acidophilus*, *L. rhamnosus* GG has been investigated, too. Peter Cadieux and his colleagues at the Canadian Research and Development Centre for Probiotics at the Lawson Health Research Institute in London, Ontario, in collaboration with associates at the University of Western Ontario, investigated various *Lactobacillus* strains and their effectiveness in controlling genitourinary infections, including candidal vaginitis. They found that the GG strain of *L. rhamnosus* was ineffective for preventing urinary tract infections (UTIs). They turned their attention to the GR-1 strain of *L. rhamnosus* and to *L. fermentum* RC-14 to ascertain whether these strains had any anti-yeast or antiviral properties. Women with genitourinary tract infections were given the GR-1 and RC-14 strains in capsules. After fourteen days, the participants showed significantly higher colonization levels of one or both of these organisms than those given the GG strain. Consistently, both GR-1 and RC-14 inhibited the growth of *C. albicans*. Culture fluid from the two strains killed vesicular stomatitis virus (VSV), an acute viral disease in farm animals, and the adenovirus, which infects the upper respiratory tract in humans. These viruses were killed within ten minutes.

Cadieux and his colleagues suggested that all probiotic strains of *Lactobacillus*, even of the same species, do not necessarily act similarly at the same site. In the researchers' studies, the anti-yeast activity of the two effective strains of *Lactobacillus* brought long-term benefits to more than fifty women in the study who used weekly vaginal *Lactobacillus* therapy for up to one year. They had few recurrent episodes—far fewer than would be expected if left untreated or treated ineffectively. Also, the researchers suggested that the potent antiviral activity demonstrated by the two strains of *Lactobacillus* might explain, in part, the reduced risk of women to acquire sexually transmitted diseases, including HIV, if the women are colonized by lactobacilli. The concluding recommendation was "given that women may have abnormal vaginal flora at many times during their menstrual cycle, the ability to restore a lactobacilli-dominated flora using self-care products such as selected probiotics could prove helpful."

ADVANTAGES OF PROBIOTICS OVER DRUGS

Biotherapeutic agents such as *L. acidophilus* and other strains have advantages over the commercial drugs used for *C. albicans* and other genitourinary infections. Production of the biotherapeutics is relatively simple and inexpensive. The agents have low risk. The use of biotherapeutic agents to treat infectious diseases may well become an important model for research and development by the pharmaceutical industry.

CHAPTER 10

Yogurt and Structures, Organs, and Systems

The possible health benefits of yogurt for various structures, organs, and systems of the body are underinvestigated. Results from relatively few studies indicate that this unchartered area is worthy of further explorations.

PROBIOTICS AND BONE HEALTH

Bone resorption is the loss of minerals, especially calcium, from the bone. Yogurt may enhance bone health by strengthening it, and by retarding bone loss. Frequently, postmenopausal women have bone resorption, followed by bone fragility, fractures, breakages, and falls.

Can the consumption of yogurt, a high-calcium food, help reverse bone resorption? Robert P. Heaney, M.D., and his team from the Osteoporosis Research Center at Creighton University in Omaha, Nebraska, attempted to answer that question. They enrolled twenty-nine postmenopausal women with habitually low calcium intakes, who showed signs of bone resorption. The women were not on estrogen therapy, which helps bone absorb calcium, nor did they use calcium supplements. In the study, three servings of yogurt were substituted for a nutritionally poor snack that the women had been consuming in their daily diet. Within seven to ten days, the study showed that bone resorption can be reduced rapidly with improved calcium intake. Also, the satiety effect of the yogurt substantially improved the overall quality of the diet. These changes were achieved readily in older women merely by daily yogurt consumption.

Risk of bone fractures in younger people, too, may be lessened with lactic acid-containing dairy products such as yogurt. A component in the whey, known as milk basic protein (MBP), has been investigated by different groups of Japanese researchers.

One group, led by Yasuhiro Toba and reported in 2000, began with laboratory experiments with ovariectomized female rats. (The procedure is the equivalent of surgically removed ovaries in women, with the resulting deficiency of estrogen production.) The rats were fed MBP to assess bone strength and bone resorption. After seventeen weeks of feeding, there was a significant retention of bone strength and lessening of bone loss in the rats receiving a high MBP-supplemented diet.

Another group, led by Seiichiro Aoe and reported in 2001, conducted clinical trials with thirty-three young Japanese women, averaging nearly twenty-nine years of age. The women were fed daily a lactic acid beverage with or without 40 milligrams (mg) of whey-derived MBP for six months. Their bone mineral density, measured in the left heel bone, was significantly greater in the group fed the beverage containing MBP than in the group fed the untreated beverage.

In a followup study, conducted by Toba and his group and reported in 2001, bone benefits from MBP were found by giving a far higher dose for a shorter time period. The team gave thirty young men, averaging about thirty-six years of age, a beverage similar to the one used by the Aoe team, but supplemented with whey-derived MBP at a daily dose of 300 mg, and for a brief period of only sixteen days. Then, the researchers measured biochemical markers, which showed reduced bone loss and increased bone formation with the high dosage over a short time. There was no noticeable effect on urinary calcium, which would indicate retention or loss.

Then, in another followup study by the Aoe team, reported in 2005, thirty-two postmenopausal women, averaging about fifty years of age, were given a similar whey-derived beverage containing the same level of MBP (40 mg) as the team had given to the younger women in the earlier study. Also, the new study lasted a similar length of time (six months) as the older study. The women in the study were not being treated with hormone replacement therapy. After six months, the study showed that the women who had received the MBP-supplemented beverage achieved greater gain in bone mineral density in the lumbar area of the spine than the women who had received the unsupplemented beverage.

These various studies suggest that whey-derived MBP is potentially beneficial to promote bone health and arrest bone loss associated with declining estrogen in women. At present, the osteoactive constitutents in MBP are unidentified. It is suggested that there may be an interplay with several peptides and growth factors. Laboratory studies suggest that in human digestion, an orally active osteoactive peptide may be created. Further investigation is needed to understand the beneficial role of MBP as an addition to calcium- and lactic acid-containing foods such as yogurt.

PROBIOTICS AND ORAL HEALTH

As early as 1964, *Lactobacillus acidophilus* was shown to be helpful in treating herpetic gingivostomatitis, an acute inflammatory infection of the mouth and gums. Jerome Lichtenstein and his associates at the Elmhurst General Hospital in New York treated eleven patients who manifested this disease with a viable strain of *L. acidophilus* and whole-milk products. According to Lichtenstein's enthusiastic report, the results were "sufficiently dramatic to warrant reporting, and indicate the desirability of further, more definite studies. Within twelve hours, all patients reported relief of pain; in twenty-four hours, eating without difficulty was restored; and after seventy-two hours, the patients were lesion free."

Lactobacillus rhamnosus GG, mentioned last chapter for its value against vaginal yeast infections, is also beneficial in the oral cavity. (It is also effective against diarrhea, atopic dermatitis, ulcerative colitis, and other health conditions.) Supplementation with *L. rhamnosus* GG may help prevent dental caries in children, possibly by reducing cariogenic bacteria in the mouth. In a study led by L. Nase, reported in 2001, 594 children, one to six years of age, were randomly assigned to drink milk supplemented with *L. rhamnosus* GG or unsupplemented milk. After seven months, the incidence of dental caries was 49 percent lower in the group of children who had consumed the supplemented milk than in the control group. The beneficial effects of *L. rhamnosus* GG were most pronounced in children three to four years of age. Their mouths contained lesser amounts of the cariogenic bacterium, *Streptococcus mutans*.

PROBIOTICS AND EYE HEALTH

The relationship of yogurt and eye health is a sensationalized but instructive story. It began in the 1950s with two scientists from Johns Hopkins University in Baltimore, Maryland who were studying a stomach disorder, not an eye disorder. A psychobiologist Carl P. Richter and an opthalmologist James R. Duke were studying the cause of paroxysmal peritonitis, a stomach disorder common to certain Mediterranean populations of Armenians, Jews, and Arabs. The scientists searched for any factors shared in the lives of these people. Fermented milk, especially yogurt, formed a large part of the dietary intake of all these people. It appeared to be the common denominator. A number of patients among these groups had symptoms of gastrointestinal allergy. When milk was eliminated from their diets, the symptoms subsided. Richter and Duke decided to research yogurt's effect on health.

Their initial test was with four rats. The animals were given access to separate containers of the usual stock feed, yogurt, and water. All four rats consumed large amounts of yogurt, and greatly reduced their intake of the stock feed. They drank little water. Each of the rats grew at a normal rate, displayed normal activity, and remained in what appeared to be excellent health. The researchers began to wonder if yogurt could be considered as "a perfect food."

Attempting to answer this question, the researchers kept another group of four rats on an exclusive diet of yogurt and water, and excluded the stock feed. These rats, too, ate large amounts of yogurt, but drank little water. They did not appear to miss the stock feed. Their estrous cycles were regular. They mated, and produced normal healthy litters. They nursed and nurtured the offspring until weaning. A third generation of rat pups was born. By then, the experiment appeared to demonstrate that yogurt was a complete food. However, the unanticipated occurred.

Quizzical Findings

By chance, the scientists noted that all four original rats had developed mature cataracts in both eyes. The gradual changes in the lenses of the animals had escaped notice because the researchers had not been looking for them. The finding was especially intriguing because no rat in the forty-year-old colony from which they had been selected had ever developed a cataract spontaneously on stock feed.

The finding posed several questions. How long does it take for an all-yogurt diet to produce changes in the lens that precede cataract formation? What are the clinical features of these cataracts compared with cataracts produced by other experimental methods? Most importantly, what factor(s) in the all-yogurt diet was (were) responsible for the lens changes?

In an attempt to answer these questions, Richter and Duke arranged for another test, using twenty-six rats. At the beginning of the experiment, the rats were 34 to 221 days of age. Again, the rats were given an all-yogurt diet. None of the rats, even those that were observed for more than a year, showed any obvious abnormalities that would have indicated malnutrition. There was no loss of hair, dermatitis, defects of teeth, signs of diarrhea, incoordinate gait, or convulsive movements. The sole adverse finding was cataract formation.

Except for the cataract formation, it would appear that yogurt was a fairly complete food. There are no known foods on which rats or other animals, including humans, can exist in a healthy state for any length of time if one food is the sole component of the diet. Yet the all-yogurt diet had not induced malnutrition. Autopsies of the experimental animals showed no abnormal cell changes. Blood had the normal number of red and white cells. Sodium and potassium concentrations in the blood were normal. Calcium and phosphorus concentrations were slightly elevated, probably because milk is a good source of both minerals. But why did the yogurt induce cataracts?

The researchers noted that the onset of lens changes in the rats had appeared to be related to the age of the animals at the time when the diet was started. The lens changes seemed to appear more quickly in the younger animals than in the older animals. At the beginning of the study, the six youngest rats were 34 days old. They developed the first striae (streaks) that signaled the beginning of cataract formation after twenty-eight to forty-two days. At the beginning of the test, the six oldest rats were 221 days old. They developed the first striae after sixty-eight to eighty-three days.

Seeking further to learn the cause of the cataracts, the researchers examined how the yogurt was manufactured, by analyzing the milk's composition, especially its galactose content. Earlier, H. S. Mitchell and W. M. Dodge had reported that cataracts could be induced in rats at a level of 22 percent galactose in the diet (*J Nutr*, 1935). Traditionally, yogurt is produced from whole milk. The lactose breaks down into glucose and galactose. Whole milk contains only 14.4 percent galactose, and yogurt made from whole milk contains only 14.2 percent galactose. These values are well below the 22 percent level noted by Mitchell and Dodge.

In having the yogurt composition analyzed, Richter and Duke were astounded to find that the commercial yogurt they had used in their experiments had a far higher galactose content: from 22 to 24 percent, levels within the range found by Mitchell and Dodge to induce cataracts in rats. Indeed, the analysis of the yogurt used in the study accounted for the cataracts in their rats. Although the finding answered their puzzlement, it raised another question. Why did the commercial yogurt made from milk have much more galactose than is contained in the milk?

Richter and Duke discovered that commercial yogurt manufactured in the United States is no longer simply the product of fermentative action on whole milk. Frequently, most of the butterfat removal results in milk with relatively more carbohydrate, and thus, more galactose. Lacking butterfat, the liquid is thin and watery, as mentioned earlier in the discussion of lactose intolerance (pages 48–50). In order to improve the consistency of reduced- or non-fat dairy products, including yogurt, processors may add skim milk powder, which further increases the caloric percentage of galactose in the yogurt. Thus, the commercial procedure used to make yogurt is responsible for the high galactose content in many yogurts, especially in reduced- or non-fat yogurts.

Richter and Duke had solved the puzzle. The high galactose in the commercial yogurt was the culprit in the rats' cataract formation. In experiments, cataracts intentionally induced in rats by galactose are clinically indistinguishable from those induced by feeding rats high galactose-containing yogurt.

Not All Yogurts Are Alike

Fifteen years after Richter and Duke had completed their studies, their findings were published in *Science* in 1970. Immediately, the findings were picked up by many newspapers and magazines in a distorted and sensationalized manner. Headlines warned that yogurt was a dangerous food. This hysteria can only be understood within the context of the period. It was a time when it was commonplace to ridicule "natural foods." Anyone who favored basic foods over the highly processed ones that were proliferating, was regarded as a lunatic fringer who wore long hair, was clad in Birkenstocks, and was sustained by blackstrap molasses, brewer's yeast, seaweed, and—yes—yogurt.

By 1970, Richter and Duke could not even remember which brands of yogurt they had used in their experiments. They were concerned about individuals who might depend on commercial yogurt as their mainstay. But, they concluded in their comments that appeared in the *Journal of the American Medical Association* that a normal day-to-day consumption of commercial or homemade yogurt, as part of the diet, was without risk.

Only under extreme conditions of use might yogurt produce cataracts in humans. In this connection, it is of interest to note that in areas of India, where defatted yogurt forms a large part of the diet, the incidence of cataracts is very high.

Discussions of various aspects of the galactose issue followed the Richter and Duke report. Margarita Nagy, from the American Medical Association's Department of Food and Nutrition, pointed out that yogurt is only a small fraction of the human diet. Also, the rat's metabolic system

Intestinal Flora and Obesity

Intestinal flora may play a role in regulating body weight. Two types of beneficial bacteria, Bacteroidetes and Firmicutes, reside in the gut. The ratio of these two bacteria appears to be important in determining an individual's propensity for obesity. A research team led by Ruth Ley at the Center for Genome Sciences and the Genome Sequencing Center at Washington University in St. Louis, Missouri, examined these bacteria. Experiments with genetically obese mice and their lean littermates, as well as clinical trials with obese and lean human volunteers, showed an association between obesity and an increased abundance of Firmicutes compared with Bacteroidetes. Furthermore, in humans, the relative abundance of Bacteroidetes increased as obese individuals lost weight, and the increase correlated significantly to weight loss but not to total caloric intake.

The researchers performed biochemical and genomic analyses of the gut microbes in obese and lean mice. They found that the microbial genomes of the bacteria found in obese mice were amply supplied with gene-encoding enzymes that break down otherwise indigestible food. This effect resulted in an increased capacity to obtain caloric energy from the diet. This trait could be transferred to germ-free mice receiving microbes from the guts of obese mice. The formerly germ-free mice experienced a significantly greater increase in total body fat without increased food consumption than the germ-free mice receiving microbes from lean mice. The researchers concluded that the results "identify the gut microbiota as an additional contributing factor to the pathophysiology of obesity" (*Nature*, 2006).

differs from that of humans. The rat has an enzymatic deficiency that does not allow it to tolerate lactose or galactose. Most humans have an adequate supply of the enzyme, except for those people who have a fairly rare congenital deficiency known as galactocemia and who must avoid foods high in galactose.

We can draw lessons from the experiments of Richter and Duke. A mono diet of any one food is unwise. There is wisdom in the age-old practice of choosing a wide variety of foods. As part of the diet, yogurt makes a good contribution. The findings of Richter and Duke should be viewed as a condemnation of present food-processing practices, rather than falsely blaming a wholesome food. This feature was the real story, yet it was totally overlooked in the sensational reportings.

PROBIOTICS AND CARDIOVASCULAR HEALTH

An early study from 1965 discounted the role of yogurt in reducing cholesterol. Researchers Beatrice L. Gold and Paul Samuel reported on their attempt to reduce cholesterol levels in nine patients. Six of the patients had unusually high levels of cholesterol and three (the controls) had normal levels. The patients were given one to two cups of yogurt daily for six to twenty-two weeks. The yogurt failed to influence serum cholesterol. The study failed to specify the amount of butterfat in the yogurt, which might have been a critical factor.

Following that study, more recent ones have demonstrated that yogurt can reduce cholesterol, or that yogurt can increase the so-called good HDL (high-density lipoprotein) cholesterol and reduce the so-called bad LDL (low-density lipoprotein) cholesterol.

George V. Mann at Vanderbilt University Medical School, Nashville, Tennessee, in behalf of the National Heart and Lung Institute of the National Institutes of Health, had conducted extensive cholesterol tests for a decade in Africa. Mann was assisted by Anne Spoerry of the African Medical Research Foundation. At first, the project of Mann and Spoerry was to test the effects of surfactants on blood cholesterol. Surfactants are a widely used class of food additives. They permit oil and water to mix more readily, and were appearing in many processed foods such as commercial mayonnaise, ice cream, baked goods, and chocolate, as well as in nonfood consumer items such as detergents.

In earlier studies with rabbits, monkeys, and dogs, Mann found that blood cholesterol levels of the animals rose when surfactants were present in the animals' rations at levels commonly used in American foodstuffs. It was important to learn whether the surfactants were raising cholesterol levels in humans.

Probiotics Reduce Cholesterol Levels

Mann returned to East Africa to test this observation in humans. He chose to work with a group of Masai tribesmen, tall and slender nomadic cattle herders in southern Kenya and northern Tanzania. Mann had already studied the Masai because they were known to be unusually resistant to coronary diseases despite their diet high in animal fats and cholesterol. Their daily diet consisted of about a gallon of fermented whole milk as a kind of homemade yogurt, and with a weekly feast of meat and animal blood. Their cholesterol intake from foods was nearly twice the amount recommended at that time for Americans by the American Heart Association. Yet the Masai's cholesterol levels were far lower than those of average American adult males.

Because the Masai had no exposure to surfactants, and with their very low blood cholesterol levels, Mann felt that they would be excellent candidates in a carefully conducted study to test the effects of the surfactants on their cholesterol. Mann chose twenty-four young Masai men and divided them into two groups. One group ate their customary yogurt to which a surfactant was added. The other group (the control) ate untreated yogurt. Because the food was supplied freely, the men kept requesting more. Soon, they were consuming twice their normal intake of yogurt. Not surprisingly, the men began to gain weight. Mann was concerned because weight gain is a known factor that can raise cholesterol levels and cause cardiovascular problems. Mann decided it would be ethical to stop the study.

When Mann measured the cholesterol levels of the men, he was surprised. At the end of the incomplete study, the blood cholesterol levels in both groups had *dropped* significantly from the levels measured at the beginning of the study. In fact, the more yogurt the men had consumed and the more weight they had gained, the greater was the drop in blood cholesterol! Mann concluded that the dramatic drop must have resulted from the body's own mechanism for adjustments. If too little cholesterol is consumed from foods, the body adapts and produces more cholesterol to meet the body's needs. Adequate cholesterol is essential for several vital functions, including cell membrane production.

After Mann finished his study with the Masai, he wondered if the findings were applicable to Americans, too. He studied twelve adult Americans who were given two liters (a little more than two quarts) of yogurt daily, with a sufficient amount of their usual foods to maintain normal weight. Mann found that the results were similar to those of the Masai. Yogurt lowered their cholesterol levels, but unfermented milk did not. Mann suggested that Americans could achieve cholesterol reduction, as did the Masai, by daily yogurt consumption.

Mann proposed that the yogurt bacteria produce some substance (probably a small fatty acid) that blocks cholesterol production in the liver. Although Mann credited yogurt consumption with cholesterol reduction, he also emphasized that it was not the sole factor that protected the Masai against cardiovascular diseases. He noted that, as nomads, the average young Masai walked up to twenty-five miles daily, and even the elderly men walked seven or eight miles daily. Mann declared that the typical Masai was as physically fit as a trained American athlete.

Mann's findings regarding yogurt were strengthened further in 1978 by a food scientist, Thomas Richardson, at the University of Wisconsin at Madison. Richardson noted that research indicated that there were factors in fermented milk which prevented the buildup of cholesterol in blood. Yogurt consumption reduced cholesterol levels.

The following year, a joint study by the University of California, Los Angeles (UCLA) General Hospital and the College of Medicine at Penn State University, at Hershey, showed that serum cholesterol could be reduced by 5 to 10 percent in a group of healthy adults by eating yogurt for only one week. Subsequent to that finding, fifty-four volunteers were studied for twelve weeks, during which time their diet was supplemented with three cups (240 ml) of yogurt or milk daily at varying times each day. The participants kept food diaries, and they were encouraged to maintain their regular diets and exercise patterns. They showed changes after following the regimen. Yogurt supplementation reduced their total serum cholesterol levels significantly, but did not affect their serum triglycerides, nor did it affect their weight. (Triglycerides are neutral fats that are the usual storage form of fats in humans.) A 2-percent butterfat milk in the control group also lowered the serum cholesterol level, but by an amount that was less statistically significant.

According to researchers at Penn State, the constituents in milk that lower cholesterol are still unknown. Milk has some 3,000 clearly identified compounds. Among them are at least 176 complex fatty acids. Some researchers have suggested that lactose, calcium, and a water-soluble complex acid might be the cholesterol-production inhibitors. Other researchers have thought that orotic acid was the inhibitor. But other researchers proposed that cholesterol-blocking compounds might be substances with higher molecular weight than orotic acid, and not be a standard fat or protein. They hypothesized that it might be a substance that would block the cholesterol synthesis at a different step than orotic acid, which acts on the second of the body's twenty-six-step process in the cholesterol synthesis chain. The puzzle remains unsolved.

In 1981, additional support was given to previous findings by researchers at the Food Science and Technology Department, University of Nebraska at Lincoln, who showed that cultured dairy products have some special nutritional properties. Supplementing diets of both humans and laboratory animals with cultured dairy products reduced serum cholesterol levels in both groups.

Does daily consumption of yogurt keep cholesterol levels low? Perhaps not. The July–August 1984 issue of the *Journal of Food Science* reported a clinical trial with ten adult males. Their customary diets were modified by adding 681 grams of yogurt daily (approximately three cups) throughout three periods of fourteen to twenty-one days. A different set of select strains was used to culture the yogurt. The inclusion of yogurt into the daily diet significantly reduced total serum cholesterol 10 to 12 percent. However, after continuous yogurt consumption, serum cholesterol levels returned to the levels at the beginning of the study. Serum triglycerides and the proportions of serum lipoproteins (fats attached to protein) were not influenced significantly by yogurt consumption. This study yielded contradictory results to others.

It was learned that certain strains of *L. acidophilus* attack bile acids, and cleave off an amino acid from a steroid bile salt. Because bile salts are synthesized in the body from cholesterol, animal scientists, led by Stanley Gilliland at Oklahoma State University in Stillwater, showed that under conditions that exist in the gastrointestinal (GI) tract, certain strains of *L. acidophilus* absorb cholesterol. In one study, Gilliland and his team fed pigs a diet containing a gram of pure crystalline cholesterol. This amount of cholesterol was considered to be enough to raise the animals' normal serum cholesterol levels. Animals given the milk containing the *L. acidophilus* gained a serum cholesterol concentration of only 9 milligrams (mg) per deciliter (dl) of blood, which was half as much as the 18 mg/dl increase experienced by the pigs given milk without the addition of *L. acidophilus*. Gilliland and his colleagues found that *L. acidophilus* varies among strains in its ability to assimilate cholesterol. Also, the bacterium has evolved with a certain host specificity. For example, strains cultured in pigs do not thrive in humans, and vice versa. However, the researchers found at least one cholesterol-active strain that is specific to humans. The finding was strengthened by studies elsewhere, demonstrating that cholesterol levels in human infants could be reduced by feeding them formulas supplemented with *L. acidophilus*.

Although Gilliland and his team used pigs for their experiments, their findings may be applicable to humans. Pigs make good animal models to extrapolate to humans because their intestinal and circulatory systems are similar to those of humans; the systems of rodents are less similar.

More recent research has shown the effects of long-term daily yogurt consumption on serum cholesterol. G. Kiebling led a team that found probiotic cultures in yogurt increased serum HDL cholesterol levels and decreased the ratio of LDL to HDL cholesterol levels. The yogurt chosen for the study had been cultured with *Streptococcus thermophilus* and *Lactococcus lactis*, and contained 3.5 percent butterfat. The researchers supplemented the yogurt with one of several strains of *L. acidophilus* for seven weeks in random order. The participants in the study, twenty-nine healthy women from nineteen to fifty years of age, consumed 300 grams (approximately one and a third cups) daily of the supplemented yogurt for seven weeks. After that time period, the women were switched to regular yogurt (the control), for another seven weeks. Intake of the supplemented yogurt as well as the regular yogurt had no significant effect on their average serum LDL levels. But both yogurts showed a significant *increase* in their average HDL levels, and a significant *decrease* in their average ratio of LDL to HDL cholesterol levels. Therefore, the intake of yogurt showed favorable results with cholesterol.

One can speculate about these studies using cultured milk to reduce cholesterol. Some of the studies fail to specify the butterfat content of the yogurt, or whether the product was made from whole or reduced-fat milk. Because the butterfat content was shown to be a crucial factor in the Richter and Duke findings of cataract formation in rats, discussed earlier (see pages 66–68), this feature may distort some of the findings regarding yogurt's ability to reduce cholesterol in humans.

PROBIOTICS AND BLOOD PRESSURE

Normal blood pressure is a component of cardiovascular health. Many Americans have hypertension (high blood pressure), and some have hypotension (low blood pressure). These conditions, especially hypertension, if untreated, can lead to major health problems, including stroke. Frequently, drugs are prescribed, and some dietary recommendations are given. Patients generally are told to adhere to a low-sodium diet, and to eat a generous amount of potassium-rich fruits such as bananas, oranges, and berries. Usually, the dietary recommendations fail to include yogurt. Yet, recent research appears to indicate that fermented milk may be beneficial in lowering high blood pressure.

In Finland, a dairy company, Valio, in 2000 launched a new cultured milk product, Evolus, with a claim that the product could lower blood pressure. Evolus is flavored with bilberry (a berry that somewhat resembles the American blueberry), and contains a special *Lactobacillus* strain that produces bioactive peptides in the milk. (Peptides are compounds that, upon hydrolysis, yield two or more amino acids: polypeptides yield more than two.) Valio conducted laboratory studies with SHR rats, a strain bred to develop high blood pressure. Evolus was tested against traditionally cultured milk, water, pure peptides, and a Japanese product Ameal S, made by Calpis, and reported to be similar to Evolus. Of all the substances fed the rats, Evolus had the strongest antihypertensive effect on the animals. The amount of lowered blood pressure in the rats by Evolus was judged to be statistically significant.

Following the animal studies, Valio conducted double-blind placebo-controlled clinical studies with humans. The participants were individuals with moderately high blood pressure but who were not taking any antihypertensive medication. A daily dose of 1.5 dl of Evolus (approximately two-thirds cup) decreased blood pressure about 5 to 10 percent in the participants. Valio reported that "the product will give an excellent support for the dietary therapy of a person with high blood pressure."

In the United States, Chr. Hansen, a supplier of nutraceuticals, headquartered in Hoersholm, Denmark, has been researching lactic acid bacteria as substances that can reduce blood pressure. Animal studies conducted by the company demonstrated that their culture, named Cardio-4, reduced high blood pressure in experimental animals. In 2005, Chr. Hansen announced that it had filed for a patent on the culture, and expected that the product would be available in supermarkets in a few years.

Probiotics Target ACE Inhibitor

Angiotensin is a polypeptide formed in blood plasma. The angiotensin-converting enzyme (ACE) regulates blood pressure. The inactive form, angiotensin I, is acted upon by a peptide enzyme, peptidase, to make angiotensin II, the active form, which is a vasopressor (vasoconstrictor). ACE is a common target for hypertensive medications.

ACE inhibitors have antihypertensive effects. Peptides derived from milk protein can have ACE-inhibiting characteristics, and therefore, also may have antihypertensive effects. A study led by Leena Seppo reported in 2003 that fermented milk supplemented with two bioactive tripeptides (peptides that contain three amino acids) in *Lactobacillus helveticus* LBK-16H, used daily were found to help lower blood pressure in individuals who are hypertensive. Seppo and her team conducted a clinical trial with thirty-nine hypertensive patients from thirty to sixty-two years of age. The two groups were closely matched. At the beginning of the study, their mean systolic and diastolic blood pressures were 155 and 97 mm Hg (millimeters of mercury) respectively in the first group, and 152 and 96 mm Hg respectively in the second group. One group received approximately two-thirds cup (150 ml) of fermented milk supplemented with the *Lactobacillus* strain containing the bioactive tripeptides; the other group was given unsupplemented fermented milk. The participants took weekly blood pressure measurements at home with automatic blood pressure recorders. During the study, blood pressure levels decreased in both groups, but the decreases were significantly more in the group consuming the supplemented fermented milk than in the control group. At the end of the twenty-one-week study, the average systolic and diastolic blood pressure readings had declined by 6.7 and 3.6 mm Hg respectively in the test group, and 3.6 and 1.9 mm Hg respectively in the control group. The test group had achieved nearly twice the decline in blood pressure readings as the control group. The researchers had demonstrated that fermented milk can lower blood pressure, and if bioactive peptides are added to fermented milk, blood pressure can be lowered even more.

Another study with fermented milk containing *L. helveticus* demonstrated its ability to lower blood pressure in hypertensives. A team led by T. Jauhiainen reported their findings in the *American Journal of Hypertension* (2005). The researchers gave ninety-four hypertensive patients who were not on antihypertensive medication either a fermented milk supplemented with *L. helveticus*, two types of tripeptides, and potassium, calcium, and magnesium, or a fermented milk without *L. helveticus* or the tripeptides, and with lower levels of the added minerals. The two tripeptides used were the same as those used in the Seppo studies, previously discussed. The tripeptides had been found to reduce blood pressure in animal experiments. After daily consumption of a glass of the supplemented fermented milk for ten weeks, the participants benefited. Those on the highly supplemented drink showed an average 4 mm Hg decrease in systolic pressure and an average of almost 2 mm Hg decrease in diastolic pressure. The decreases were not as good as those in the Seppo study, but the participants were in the Jauhiainen study only half as long as the participants in the Seppo study. Perhaps over a longer time period, the decreases might have been greater. The Jauhiainen team attributed the beneficial results from the action of the tripeptides to their ability to inhibit ACE.

PROBIOTICS AND CELL HEALTH

Because the beneficial bacteria in cultured milk display antimicrobial activity, it is reasonable to expect that they support cellular health. There have been spasmodic attempts to demonstrate the antitumor activity of these bacteria, but to date there has been no comprehensive program to explore the full range of their potential. The following citations represent some milestones.

Probiotics Reduce Cancer-Cell Formation

The work of Ivan Bogdanov and his colleagues, Peter Popchristov and Luben Marinov, all from the Scientific Research Institute for Anticancer Antibodies, of the Academy of Sciences in Bulgaria, was reported in *Medical World News* (Sept 28, 1962). The researchers had implanted 455 mice with sarcoma 180 (Sa 180), a transplantable malignant tumor commonly used to test animals with antitumor agents. Then, they injected the mice with 0.5 to 1 ml of filtered *Lactobacillus bulgaricus*, in the seventh, eighth, ninth, or tenth day after the implant. Usually Sa 180 induces fatal malignant tumors such as sarcomas and ascites. Sa 180 is regarded as an incurable tumor. However, due to the potent antitumor activity of *L. bulgaricus*, 136 of the 455 mice developed tumors but remained cancer free. Seven days after the injection, the lesions in the 136 mice darkened, necrotized, dehydrated, shrank, and dropped off. The remaining ulcerations healed and eventually the scars were covered over by hair. The cancer-free mice remained healthy throughout a 200-day followup period. All of the mice treated with Sa 180, but not injected with *L. bulgaricus*, died.

Attempts to induce tumors in the cancer-free mice by another Sa 180 transplant failed. Apparently, the mice had developed immunity.

Khem M. Shahani, professor of food science, University of Nebraska at Lincoln, had worked for years on cultured milk products. He noted that yogurt had been reported to have potent antitumor activity. Shahani and his colleagues reported on their investigations in the *Journal of the National Cancer Institute* in the March 1973 issue. The Shahani team transplanted tumors into two groups of mice that had been maintained on normal diets. The test group was given yogurt mixed with their drinking water. The control group was given plain water. After eight days, the yogurt-fed mice showed an average of 28 percent less cell proliferation than the control group. The mice in the control group showed rapid tumor growth for six days, and then the tumor growth leveled off. When interviewed, Shahani reported that yogurt has natural antitumor properties that may help retard or prevent the onset of disease. But he cautioned that to say that all yogurts have such qualities is unjustified. The potency varies from product to product.

Probiotics Confer Additional Antitumor Effects

L. acidophilus may play a beneficial role in one of the most common and potent types of cancer: colon or large bowel cancer. It is thought that dietary factors play an important role. High intakes of fat and meat have been associated with colon cancer. Barry Goldin and Sherwood L. Gorbach, both from the Tufts University School of Medicine in Boston, substituted meat for grain in the diet of laboratory rats. The levels of three enzymes involved in forming cancer-inducing substances in the GI tract rose sharply. When the feed was supplemented with *L. acidophilus*, the levels of all three enzymes declined. Two of the enzymes decreased to the level found in the grain-fed animals, and the third enzyme dropped slightly. Goldin and Gorbach reported their findings in the March 1977 issue of the *Cancer Journal*.

Obviously, the potential health benefits of cultured milk products are of great interest to the dairy industry. Through its journals and periodicals, it publishes reports on experiments that demonstrate the antitumor activity of beneficial bacteria in yogurt. *Dairy Research Digest* in March

1983 noted a study of male Swiss mice, implanted with Ehrlich tumors and then injected with components of yogurt starter culture. The mice could consume as much yogurt as they wanted for seven consecutive days. Tumor cell proliferation was inhibited by 25 to 32 percent. Injected cultures inhibited tumor cell proliferation in direct proportion to the number of starter culture cells implanted.

The October 1983 issue of *Dairy Research Digest* reported on the antileukemic effects in mice from fermentation products of *L. bulgaricus.* The milk was fermented for seven days with a special strain of the bacterium, and then was injected into leukemic-induced mice. Results showed antileukemic effects of the *L. bulgaricus.*

The January 1984 issue of *Dairy Research Digest* reported on the antitumor effects of *Lactobacillus helveticus* var. *jugurti* and its physicochemical properties.

By the 1990s, papers were presented at the annual meetings of the Institute of Food Technology (IFT) on antimutagens in yogurt. IFT's *1994 Book of Abstracts* has a summary of a paper presented by the lead researcher, Sudarshan R. Nadathur, Department of Food Science and Technology at Oregon State University in Corvallis, on the production of antimutagens in yogurt by lactic acid bacteria. The following year, the same team of researchers summarized their work to identify the antimutagens in yogurt. The summary of their paper appeared in IFT's *1995 Book of Abstracts.*

Despite the lack of any comprehensive program to explore the full range of cell protection offered by bacteria in cultured milk, certain findings are well established. It is recognized that these probiotics have the ability to suppress

- mutagenicity in cells (activity that induces genetic mutations in the cells)

- genotoxicity in cells (activity that induces genetic mutations in the cells)

- carcinogenicity in cells (activity that induces cellular changes and leads to cancer)

- cell growth and differentiation of tissue culture cells

- aberrant crypt foci (precancerous formations in recessed areas in the colonic tissue of animals)

- various tumors in mice, found in organs such as the liver and colon, and in the mammary gland

- activity of certain enzymes that are involved in the conversion of pro-carcinogens (substances that enhance cancer development) with carcinogens both in humans and in laboratory animals

Now, we are ready to examine specific probiotic bactera, and the roles they play.

CHAPTER 11

Probiotic Bacteria: From Wild and Free to Controlled and Profitable

More than a decade ago, the Lactic Acid Bacteria Genome Consortium was formed. It is a collaborative effort of researchers from seven land-grant universities in different states, who are investigating eleven lactic acid bacteria and their role in the fermentation process that produces yogurt and other cultured foods. Each researcher has selected a single bacterium to study extensively. Each bacterial species has its own genetic composition, or genome. In order to understand the complexities of food-fermenting bacteria, the genome of each one needs to be sequenced. The researchers hope to learn the relationship each bacterium has with pathogenic organisms. Such knowledge may lead to advances in food preparation, as well as food safety, through improved procedures to prevent foodborne illnesses.

The consortium, collaborating with the U.S. Department of Energy's Joint Genome Institute, renowned for its work on the Human Genome Project, was able to sequence the genomes of the most important food-fermenting bacteria. The researchers used gene array technology, a useful tool to analyze the genetic expression of hundreds, or even thousands, of bacterial genes simultaneously, and under various conditions. The gene arrays allowed the researchers to find the level of expression of any one gene, and to understand how the bacterium regulates the gene in different environments, such as under heat, acidity, and salinity. Also, the researchers could inactivate certain genes related to protein metabolism and learn how the change alters the bacterium's survival or growth in certain environments.

PATENTING GENES

In recent times, there has been a trend to patent organisms that produce

Institutions Sequencing Lactic Acid Bacteria Genomes

- North Carolina State University: *Lactobacillus gasseri* and *Leuconostoc mesenteroides* subsp. *mesenteroides*
- University of California at Davis: *Oenococcus oeni*
- University of California at San Diego: *Lactobacillus brevis*
- University of Minnesota: *Bifidobacterium longum* and *Lactococcus lactis* subsp. *cremoris*
- University of Nebraska: *Streptococcus thermophilus*
- University of Wisconsin: *Lactobacillus delbrueckii* subsp. *bulgaricus*
- Utah State University: *Brevibacterium linens, Lactobacillus casei,* and *Lactococcus lactis* subsp. *cremoris*

Elsewhere, other scientists are engaged in sequencing the genomes of bacteria used for culturing milk. A team of French scientists published the genome of *Lactobacillus bulgaricus* in the *Proceedings of the National Academy of Sciences* in 2006.

Maarten van de Guchte of France's National Institute for Agricultural Research, lead author of a study, noted the ability of microorganisms to adapt to new environments. For example, originally *L. bulgaricus* may have lived on plants. The genome study showed that the bacterium contained a number of genes used to break down plant sugars. However, most of those genes appeared to be broken by mutations. Whenever this occurs, the broken genes are known as pseudogenes. They prevent the bacteria from reading their codes, and prevent them from making the corresponding proteins. The scientists were surprised to find as many as 270 pseudogenes in *L. bulgaricus,* leaving only 1,562 working genes. Also, the genome of the bacterium showed signs of having lost many other genes as well. The transformation may have begun when an ancestor of *L. bulgaricus* fell into fresh milk. Gradually, the bacterium adapted to the new environment, living in milk rather than in plants. Milk is rich in the sugar, lactose, but lacks other sugars that are found in plants. As a result, mutations destroyed *L. bulgaricus'* ability to make many of the amino acids (the building blocks of protein). Instead, it adapted to the new environment in milk. It split the milk protein and absorbed the amino acids. *L. bulgaricus* lost some genes but gained others.

yogurt, and to give them subspecies names. Typically, the two bacteria used to culture yogurt, as noted previously, are *Lactobacillus bulgaricus* and *Streptococcus thermophilus*. But subspecies now used may be designated as *Lactobacillus delbrueckii bulgaricus* and *Streptococcus salivarius thermophilus*. These are patented versions.

Joseph H. Hotchkiss, chairman of the Department of Food Science at Cornell University, Ithaca, New York, observed that such patented cultures are marketed to consumers as a way "to put more 'good' bacteria into the digestive tract." He pointed out that yogurt bacteria originally were wild organisms. (They were also free.) Before Pasteur, the organisms were propagated, in a manner of speaking, by poor hygiene. As yogurt was made, repeatedly, in the same wooden container, some culture was retained in the container and was able to inoculate each new batch of fresh milk.

After specific organisms were identified, their different strains were classified. The strains could be produced systematically, uniformly, and offer quality control. By further subdividing into designated substrains, they are patented. The bacteria are no longer wild and free. They are controlled and profitable. The patenting of probiotic bacteria has led to expanded sales. The bacteria are sold not only to food processors, but now they are manufactured also by supplement suppliers and sold to the general public as dietary supplements in capsule or powder forms, and promoted with health claims.

CONFUSING NOMENCLATURE

Formerly, subspecies' names were given to honor the individual who identified a species or strain of a microorganism. Now, the subspecies' names are more apt to designate the patent owners. Formerly, it was prestigious; presently, it is economics.

Sometimes there are name changes that result in confusion. For example, what presently is designated as *Lactobacillus rhamnosus* is known, too, as *L. rhamnosus* GG. Formerly, this bacterium was identified, as many others, simply as *Lactobacillus acidophilus*. When lactobacilli classification became designated more specifically, *L. rhamnosus* became known as *Lactobacillus casei*. Later revision classified it as *L. casei* subsp. *rhamnosus*. Still later, the bacterium attained species status of *L. rhamnosus*. Confusing? Yes! Many other *L. acidophilus* strains have been given additional identifications as a result of patenting.

What Patenting Hath Wrought

"The continual development and commercial introduction of new probiotic strains present new challenges to the scientific community. Thus, the question arises as to 'who's who' in these new cultures and what is their beta molecular taxonomy. For example, what we used to think of as *Lactobacillus acidophilus* is now known to be a mix of six different species. One is still considered *Lactobacillus acidophilus* but others such as *L. johnsonii* and *L. gasseri*, which are commonly found in humans, are considered to evoke 'acidophilus-like' probiotic properties."

—Prof. Todd Klaenhammer, North Carolina State University, quoted in
Prepared Foods Nutra Solutions, 2001

Formerly, the taxonomy of lactic acid bacteria, such as the well-known one, *Lactobacillus bulgaricus,* and less familiar ones such as *Leuconostoc* and *Pediococcus,* were based on their ability to produce lactic acid. Yet even *L. bulgaricus* formerly had been designated as *Bacillus bulgaricus.*

Newer taxonomic guidelines exclude some bacteria that formerly had been included. Various spore-bearing rods that produce lactic acid were assigned to the genus (family) of *Bacillus. Lactobacillus bifidus* was transferred to *Bifidobacterium.* Whenever a species is transferred from one genus to another, a new name or specific designation is given. Not all microbiologists may agree with the newly assigned names given by taxonomists to the microorganism. For example, the eminent microbiologist, Selman A. Waksman suggested that the *Actinomycetes* should be renamed *Streptomycetes* and unite them in a special genus, *Streptomyces.* Other microbiologists dissented, and did not believe that renaming was necessary.

At times, the lactic acid bacteria, *Enterococcus faecium,* is printed in texts by its older name, *Streptococcus faecium.* The confusion is so great that some microbiologists attempt to solve the dilemma by using the newer designation followed by the older one, such as *Lactobacillus bifidus* (*Bifidobacterium bifidum*).

A new bacterial name is accepted into bacterial nomenclature only after information about it has been established and validated by publication in a reputable scientific publication.

SINGLE STRAINS OF PROBIOTICS
AND THEIR REPORTED EFFECTS

Are probiotic strains with identified subspecies superior to the traditional ones? Do they have unique features in efficacy? The benefits of both groups appear to overlap, judging from the reported effects, which we will now examine.

Lactobacillus

Lactobacillus acidophilus, better known to the public than many other probiotic bacteria, has been found to lower fecal enzyme activity; decrease fecal mutagenicity; and to prevent radiotherapy-related diarrhea.

L. acidophilus suppresses the production of harmful substances such as ammonia, indoles, phenols, and hydrogen sulfide, all being carcinogenic and capable of damaging the liver. *L acidophilus* also suppresses the decomposition products of the six major human sources of putrefying bacteria: *Bacteroides uniformis, Acidaminococcus fermentans, Clostridium clostridiforme, Escherichia coli, Proteus vulgaris,* and *Citrobacter freundii.*

L. acidophilus La-5 is reported to balance intestinal flora, protect against travelers' diarrhea, and enhance the immune system.

Lactobacillus casei Shirota has been found helpful in preventing intestinal disturbances, balancing intestinal microflora, lowering fecal enzyme activities, and helpful in reducing the recurrence of superficial bladder cancer (that is, cancer on or near the surface).

Lactobacillus johnsonii La-1, in clinical studies, adhered to human intestinal cells, balanced intestinal flora, enhanced immunity, and proved to be a useful adjunct in *Helicobacter pylori* treatment. (*H. pylori* is a bacterial infection in the stomach, often accompanying ulcers.)

Lactobacillus reuteri is a bacterium found in breast milk that is colonized in the GI tract of healthy humans. It acts as a probiotic and produces conjugated linoleic acid (CLA), a beneficial substance also found in butterfat. *L. reuteri* can form antimicrobial substances known as reuterin and reuteri-cyclin. These substances can reduce or prevent the growth of potentially pathogenic microorganisms, including bacteria, viruses, fungi, and protozoa.

L. reuteri has been found capable of shortening the period of episodes of rotavirus-induced diarrhea. It is a patented bacterium, and commonly is sold as a dietary supplement. It is not widely available in food products, but Stonyfield Farm supplements its yogurt with *L. reuteri.*

Lactobacillus rhamnosus GG was discovered by Sherwood L. Gorbach and Barry Goldin, both at Tufts University School of Medicine: hence, the initials GG. This strain has been found to be effective in treating conditions such as rotaviral and traveler's diarrheas and intestinal upsets resulting from antibiotic treatment.

Lactobacillus sporogenes was isolated and first described in 1932 by L. M. Horowitz-Wlassowa and N. W. Nowotelnow. The discoverers selected the name for this bacterium because it produces lactic acid and bears spores. The bacterium is also known as *Bacillus coagulans*. It has been found useful against GI tract problems such as constipation and diarrhea.

Beneficial Bacteria Embedded in Drinking Straws

"The LifeTop straw, developed by BioGaia and marketed by Tetra Pak, has made its U.K. debut. Orchard Maid organic fruit yogurt drinks are packaged in a regular single-serve carton, but the interest lies in the straw attached to the side of the pack. This provides a novel yet effective way for the body to obtain probiotic cultures, as *Lactobacillus reuteri* is contained in the straw, and released only as liquid passes through it."

—Global Trends, *Prepared Foods*, September 2002

Bifidobacteria

Bifidobacterium bifidum was discovered in 1899 at the Pasteur Institute in Paris. This bacterium was found to be the predominant component in the intestinal flora of breastfed infants. The bacterium is also found in the large intestine of healthy adults, where it comprises a quarter of total gut flora. *B. bifidum* produces several specialized acids, including lactic and acetic acids. The acids inhibit pathogenic bacteria, yeasts, and some viruses. Also, *B. bifidum* can synthesize vitamin B, and improve the absorption of dietary calcium.

Reduction or lack of *B. bifidum* in the large intestine of a human indicates an unhealthy state. Oral consumption of the bacterium has been found effective in improving the intestinal environment and its flora. Dietary supplements may stimulate the immune system, help with disorders of the intestine and liver, and retard the aging process.

B. *bifidum* has long been researched in Japan, starting as early as 1950. By 1981, the Japan Bifidus Foundation was established as a central organization for bifidobacterial research. As a result, many Japanese food products were developed containing B. *bifidum*, and its use in Japan is widespread. B. *bifidum* was found to be an antitumor agent by Tomotari Mitsuoka at the Department of Biomedical Sciences, University of Tokyo. His studies published in 1990 suggest that the bacterium may have value as a cancer preventative.

B. *bifidum* has been found to recycle a toxin such as ammonia by using it as an important source of nitrogen for protein synthesis. Also, B. *bifidum* can decompose and suppress nitrosamine production in the intestine. Nitrosamines are carcinogenic compounds.

B. *bifidum* is hardy. L. M. Medina and R. Jordano, both at the University of Cordoba, Spain, reported in 1995 that B. *bifidum* can survive in commercially fermented milk, if refrigerated, for at least fifty-one days. Even after such long storage, the researchers thought that the product would still offer some dietary benefits, even though it was well past the recommended storage period (*Fd Chem News*, 1995).

Bifidobacterium lactis BB-12 was reported to promote intestinal health by adhering to the intestinal epithelial cells where it combats pathogens. The bacterium was found to be helpful in the treatment of viral diarrhea, including rotavirus, to alleviate symptoms of food allergies, and to balance the intestinal flora.

Other Useful Single Strains

Other single strains have been shown useful. Among them: B. *infantis* 35624, for irritable bowel syndrome; L. *casei* DN114-001, for immune enhancement; B. *longum* BB536, for allergies and beneficial intestinal microflora; B. *animalis* DN173-010, for normalizing intestinal transit time; L. *plantarum* 299V, for irritable bowel syndrome, and post-surgical gut health; L. *salivarius* UCC118, for inflammatory bowel disease; *Escherichia coli* Nissle 1917, for immune function and intestinal health; and *Saccharomyces cerevisiae* (*boulardii*) *lyo*, for antibiotic-induced diarrhea and infections from *Clostridium difficile*. *Streptococcus boulardii* prevents antibiotic-associated diarrhea. Also, it helps treat *Clostridium difficile*-induced colitis. Most strains of *S. thermophilus* are useful for lactose intolerance.

MIXED STRAINS OF PROBIOTICS AND THEIR REPORTED EFFECTS

Oral consumption of *L. rhamnosus* GR-1, along with *L. reuteri* RC-14, has been reported to colonize the vaginal tract and improve the therapeutic outcome for women with bacterial vaginosis.

VSL#3, consisting of eight strain blends of *S. thermophilus*, four strains of *Lactobacillus*, and three strains of *Bifidobacteria*, was reported to be useful with inflammatory bowel conditions.

The combination of *L. acidophilus* CUL60 and *B. bifidum* CUL20 has been used to reduce the toxin of *C. difficile* in feces.

L. helveticus R0052, combined with *L. rhamnosus* R0011, has been used to eradicate *H. pylori* and to alleviate diarrhea in children.

SINGLE OR MIXED STRAINS OF PROBIOTIC BACTERIA?

Traditionally, food processors focused on single strains of probiotic bacteria for specific health benefits. Now, combinations of different strains offer product developers new possibilities to explore. For example, a mixture of *L. bulgaricus*, *L. plantarum*, *S. thermophilus*, *B. longum*, *B. infantis*, and *B. breve* showed positive effects against inflammatory bowel disease and irritable bowel syndrome. Also, the mixture was reported to help prevent or alleviate radiation-associated diarrhea.

A research team led by H. M. Timmerman reviewed the functionality and efficacy of using single strains, multi-strains, and multi-species of probiotic bacteria. The multi-species mixtures showed advantages over the single strains insofar as a number of features of individual strains can be combined, provided that they are compatible. Different strains can have synergistic effects. For example, the ability of *Bifidobacterium lactis* BB-12 to adhere to intestinal cells more than doubled in the presence of *L. rhamnosus* GG or *L. bulgaricus*.

Another study, led by M. Juntunen, showed the ability of probiotic bacteria to adhere to intestinal mucus. In healthy humans, the amount of adherence differs: 34 percent of *L. rhamnosus* GG adhered, and 31 percent of *B. lactis* BB-12 adhered. But some probiotic bacteria showed far lower adhesiveness. Only 4 percent of *L. acidophilus* La-5, 3 percent of *L. paracasei*, and 1 percent of *L. casei Shirota* stayed attached to the intestinal mucus. A synergistic effect can boost the percent of adhesion by combining certain probiotic bacteria. For example, it was shown that in healthy infants adhesion of *B. lactis* BB-12, when combined with *L. rhamnosus* GG, increased from 31 percent to 39 percent adhesion.

Many claims are made about the superiority of patented over wild strains. Yet, we lack unbiased testing performed by groups other than the manufacturers who compare the two types. Similarly, many claims are made about the superiority of using mixed rather than single strains. Again, unbiased testing that compares the two approaches needs to be performed.

CHAPTER 12

Yogurt: From Plain Jane to Superstar

For many years, yogurt was a product made in American homes, mainly by people who had emigrated from countries where yogurt was a traditional staple. A smaller group of people made yogurt because they ate "health foods" and lived mostly on the East and West Coasts. Commercial yogurt was hardly available, and even the word was unknown to a vast population of Americans.

The homemade yogurt was plain, unflavored, and unadorned. It was made by saving some yogurt from each batch and adding it to the fresh milk to culture the next batch. The flavor and tartness might vary from batch to batch, due to differences in timing and temperature. Some people used a commercial culture, sent through the mail from the Rosell Institute in Montreal, Canada, a group of specialists in lactic cultures. The commercial culture gave assurance that bacteria would culture the milk and produce a uniform product.

THE YOGURT BOOM

Some enterprising immigrants began to produce commercial yogurt on a modest scale, and available to a limited area. Food processors, always eager to expand their product line, recognized that yogurt might be a profitable extension for dairy products. By the early 1970s, a boom had begun. It expanded exponentially. From the mid-1950s to the mid-1970s in the United States, yogurt sales increased 3,410 percent. By then, according to The Household Yogurt Market, a report issued by the marketing and economic research division of the United Dairy Industry Association, about 10 percent of commercial yogurt was plain; the rest were flavored and sweetened. By the end of the 1970s, a dairy trade journal, *Dairy and Ice Cream Field*, predicted a fivefold increase of yogurt consumption in the near future. Ever since, yogurt consumption has been spiraling upward. But, as nutritionist Marion Nestle wrote in her book, *What to Eat* (North Point Press, 2006), "Plain yogurt can be a nutritious and satisfying snack or accompaniment to meals, but it is easier to sell—and is more profitable—when it gets turned into a product of infinite variety and cloying sweetness."

Nestle checked the yogurt section of the refrigerated dairy cases in a medium-sized supermarket. In tallying the number of different yogurt products being offered, she rechecked her count because she could not believe the total number of different yogurt products. Her count was more than four hundred. Yet, she had a hard time to find a plain, unflavored yogurt, with nothing added except the necessary bacterial cultures.

Why such a large number of yogurt products? Nestle explained, "If you are a dairy producer and want to sell your product in a crowded supermarket, you need shelf space—and the more the better. Even if you are paying slotting fees [money paid by food distributors to grocery stores for favorable placement of foods in order to maximize sales] a carton of milk or a little cup of yogurt does not take up enough room to attract much notice. But variations on a basic product theme—'line extensions'—do. Suddenly the case is overflowing with your products, stacked one on top of another in dozens of flavors, each available as whole, low-fat, and non-fat varieties . . ."

The traditional plain yogurt, unflavored and somewhat tart, was not as appealing to the American palate as sweetened yogurt, more like a dessert.

The Exploitation of Yogurt

Yogurt producers were more interested in expanding sales than in offering health. By the mid-1970s, nearly 90 percent of all commercial yogurts were flavored with strawberry, cherry, raspberry, blueberry, peach, orange, pineapple, boysenberry, or apricot. A few flavors tentatively extended into the wild side, with lemon custard, Dutch apple, and vanilla. Later, expansions would be bolder, with flavors such as piña colada and cotton candy. Few fruit-flavored yogurts contain actual pieces of fruit. Some have sweet jam, but mainly they contain concentrated fruit juices, which are highly processed products, stripped of nutrients, but useful as flavorings. Many of these yogurts have added colors to make them appear "fruity" and thickeners to give the products some texture. The yogurts are sweetened with a number of added sugars, and some are sweetened even more by the addition of candy sprinkles, M&Ms, pieces of chocolate, or crumbles of Oreo cookies. The sweetness, described by Nestle as "cloying," masks the tartness of yogurt. Like many packaged grain cereal products, a simple commodity has been used merely as a starting point, and as a vehicle for cheap adulterative additions used to convert the product into one that will expand sales appeal. As Nestle remarked, "yogurt, it seems, has performed a marketing miracle; it is a fast-selling dairy dessert with the aura of a health food."

Yogurt was further transformed from a sweetened dessert into a junk food. By the late 1970s, the yogurt market was glutted with yogurt-containing breads, dips, salad dressings, crackers, chips, yogurt-coated pretzels, yogurt candy bars, ad infinitum.

Alexander Leaf, a cardiologist at Harvard University who was interested in longevity, visited groups of people in different areas who were reported to live for a long time. His venture in the early 1970s took him to remote areas, such as the Andes in South America, and the Caucasus in Russia. Leaf, like his predecessor Weston A. Price, author of *Nutrition and Physical Degeneration* (Price-Pottenger Foundation, 1939), found that health and longevity depended on adherence to a traditional diet, exercise, close ties with family or tribe, low stress, and a clean environment.

In studying a group of people in the Caucasus, Leaf had been told that there were many centenarians who were hale and hearty. Homemade yogurt was a mainstay in their diet. In 1973, Leaf reported his findings about different groups in an article in *National Geographic*. Leaf's findings were challenged by skeptics. Anthropologists and sociologists acknowledge that many people who do not record vital statistics tend to exaggerate their ages. They may be boastful, and their statements are unreliable.

An Old Technology in a New Package

"As early as 1966, scientists attributed the good health and longevity of the Bulgarians to the use of yogurt. Fermented milk and dairy products are not new foods. This is an old technology dressed up in a new package."

—Dr. Khem M. Shahani, professor of food science, University of Nebraska at Lincoln, interviewed by Cammy Sessa, *Virginia-Pilot Tidewater Living*, April 30, 1975

The limitations of Leaf's findings were ignored by the Dannon Company, the major commercial yogurt producer at the time. In 1975, Dannon exploited Leaf's findings about the people in the Caucasus, by funding a commercial film, used in television commercials, and stills from the film used in print advertisements. In the film, a vivacious elderly man and his equally vivacious mother, self-reported to be 89 years of age and 114 years of age, respectively, cavort in the foreground of mountains in Soviet Georgia. Also, they are shown seated, enjoying Dannon yogurt. This advertising hokum was done during a time when the Food and Drug Administration (FDA) allowed no health claims. But the implied message of the advertisement was clear: eat Dannon yogurt for vitality and longevity.

As the truth came out, the Georgian mother and son were doubtless younger than their boasts. They did not eat yogurt regularly. They certainly did not have access to Dannon yogurt. Nor did they particularly enjoy yogurt. They did become local celebrities, and the advertisements reached many people elsewhere who had never eaten yogurt.

In the last few decades, yogurt has been the top fastest-growing food product. By 2003, yogurt production in the United States had reached 2.5 billion pounds. Although this figure would seem to be a large volume, it represents only about seven pounds per capita in yearly consumption, which is low compared to yogurt consumption elsewhere. For example, in Sweden, consumption is about sixty-three pounds of yogurt per capita yearly. Other European groups consuming large amounts of yogurt include Denmark, Holland, France, and Germany. Data from elsewhere are less publicized, especially where homemade yogurt still prevails.

FROZEN YOGURT: ICE CREAM WITHOUT GUILT?

In the 1970s the early frozen yogurt products had live and active bacterial counts comparable to those in refrigerated yogurt. But, according to many industry experts, consumers rejected the tart taste in frozen yogurt. To accommodate public taste, processors reduced the acidity in their products that caused the tartness by lowering the count of live and active bacteria.

Some frozen yogurt producers would not admit that their products were competitors of ice creams. Rather, they chose to regard frozen yogurt as a "meal replacer." Such a claim has no validity. As mentioned earlier, no single food provides all the necessary nutrients required for good health.

Frozen yogurt producers ignored the question of whether the modified version of their products offered the benefits of yogurt, with live and active cultures. The modified version sold.

H. P. Hood Inc., a New England dairy with a venerable history of operating for more than a century, in 1977, launched its Frogurt Frozen Yogurt nationally, and promoted the product in six widely diverse markets. Hood competed against Dannon and Colombo in national distribution, and launched an advertising blitz on radio, outdoor billboards, and in transit subways and buses. There had been a tradition of pie-eating and doughnut-eating contests. Hood sponsored a yogurt-eating contest with Frogurt, held at D'Youville College in Buffalo, New York. The fifteen contestants consumed 288 4-ounce containers of strawberry-flavored Frogurt.

At first, Frogurt contained cultured milk, sweeteners, sodium citrate, locust bean gum, sodium carboxymethyl-cellulose, mono- and di-glycerides, and polysorbate. The sweetness had to approximate the sweetness of ice cream to be acceptable. To achieve this level of sweetness, high amounts of sweeteners were required to mask the tartness of the yogurt. Other frozen yogurts had similar formulations.

Other frozen yogurt products competed with ice cream products. The traditional popsicle was converted into Yosicle and Yoglace. In 1977, the annual retail market for frozen yogurt in the United States was estimated to be between $18 and $25 million, with a future market projected as "absolutely huge." During the same year, the annual refrigerated yogurt sales for cup yogurt had reached $350 million. The growth in sales occurred, despite the fact that only one-third of the population had ever eaten yogurt.

Marketing Frozen Yogurt

In 1975, the world's first Dannon Yogurt Store opened its doors in New York City. It featured a new soft-frozen yogurt, Danny-Yo, and nearly two dozen other yogurt specialties, including yogurt drinks, yogurt cheesecake, frozen yogurt-on-a-stick with chocolate coating, fried yogurt chips with sunflower or sesame seeds, yogurt wafers, and yogurt biscuits. The store was decorated with posters proclaiming yogurt's benefits. The poster's message was ironic, because few if any of the yogurt products sold in the store were offering any of yogurt's benefits from live active probiotic bacteria.

Frozen yogurt products, including soft-serve, began to appear everywhere. The Dannon Company (at the time, a subsidiary of Beatrice Foods Company in Chicago) began to franchise stores to sell frozen yogurt, as other stores sold ice cream.

Stores with the name "Yogurt, Yes!" became a new generation of combination yogurt/sandwich luncheon parlors. They were opened in major metropolitan cities throughout the country.

In the posh area of Bel Air, located in a popular Brentwood Village shopping area in Southern California, a "I Can't Believe *It's* Yogurt" parlor opened as a popular retail yogurt outlet. The products were soft-serve frozen yogurt. The company expanded, and became the country's second largest yogurt franchiser. Each store was expected to clear close to $5,000 a week.

The food trade journals carried numerous advertisements for equipment to make soft-serve frozen yogurt. These machines would proliferate in many restaurants, where patrons could help themselves and dispense as much frozen yogurt as they wished.

As with regular yogurt, inevitably, numerous items were added to frozen yogurt, such as health-bar chips, crumbles of peanut butter cookies, pralines, syrups, chocolate coatings, and so forth.

Frozen Yogurt More Profitable than Ice Cream

"No longer are yogurt sales limited to sophisticated tastes or health food stores. Ralph's Grocery Company, Los Angeles, tried four locations last summer where soft ice cream was replaced by soft frozen yogurt. Not only did yogurt outsell the ice cream, but profits were better."

—Howard B. Grant, *Dairy and Ice Cream Field*, October 1997

Deceptive Serving Sizes

Manufacturers prefer to have small serving sizes appear on their packages of frozen yogurt because it gives the illusion of improving the nutritional profile of the product. But it is unrealistic to suggest, as many manufacturers do, that one serving is 3 ounces (or occasionally listed as 4 ounces). In the real world, one serving is at least 6 ounces, which is double the amount on the label. The U.S. Department of Agriculture (USDA) considers about 7 ounces to be the average serving size. Even that may be unrealistic. At stores where frozen yogurt is dispensed in bowls, "small portions" are from 4 to 6 ounces, and "large portions," from 8 to 12 ounces. At the "I Can't Believe It's Yogurt" stores, mentioned earlier, the large size is 12 ounces. Many carryouts that dispense nutrition information about the frozen yogurt products list serving size in a 1-ounce portion.

Some frozen yogurts contain no live active cultures. The milk from which they are made is pasteurized, cultured, and then repasteurized, which results in the destruction of all beneficial bacteria. Tom Balmer, from the International Ice Cream Association (IICA) explained that repasteurization increases the shelflife of the product. Also, it stops the culturing process, and thereby halts further development of acidity. Because of this practice, IICA requested the FDA to require the inclusion of live active cultures as part of the definition of frozen yogurt. But, to date, there are no federal standards regarding what a product must contain in order for it to be called frozen yogurt.

By 1985, there were nearly 3,000 frozen yogurt outlets in the United States. By 1990, there were 11,000. Most of the frozen yogurt is sold as soft-serve in luncheonettes and shopping malls. In addition, the sale of hard-packed pints and quarts of frozen yogurts in American supermarkets also skyrocketed. Between 1985 and 1990, food store sales of frozen yogurt leaped from $8.3 million to a staggering $82.8 million. In recent times, annual sales have increased, albeit less dramatically.

The Critics of Frozen Yogurt

The introduction of frozen yogurt was viewed with dismay by nutritionists, dietitians, and food scientists who were aware of yogurt's beneficial properties due to the presence of live active cultures. If the probiotic bacteria in yogurt are deactivated in freezing the product, as well as the repasteurization practiced by some manufacturers, can the product really be considered to be yogurt? To this question, Manfred Kroger, at the food sciences department, Penn State University, University Park, Pennsylvania, gave a resounding "No!" Kroger said, "It cannot be denied that a sterilized, pasteurized, or even acidulated/imitation yogurt is a product of real commercial value to the milk industry. The technology and the marketplace would readily allow such a product." After this frank admission,

Kroger continued. "But the term 'yogurt' should not be allowed for such products. The term yogurt should be reserved for the living product." Kroger offered some precautionary advice. "Although some food entrepreneurs are still playing flimflam rip-off games, the dairy industry must continue its ethical history of delivering value, quality, nutrition, and dependability . . . "

Individuals who were still making homemade yogurt experienced firsthand the result of repasteurized yogurt. Formerly, they could depend on a dollop of storebought yogurt to provide them with a starter culture for their homemade yogurt. Repasteurization rendered this practice useless.

FEDERAL STANDARDS OF IDENTITY FOR YOGURT

The federal standards for regular refrigerated yogurt are weak. Although they require the presence of *Lactobacillus bulgaricus* and *Streptococcus thermophilus* for a product to be called yogurt, they fail to set the levels of these bacteria that must be present in the finished product. Because some manufacturers repasteurize yogurt, both refrigerated and frozen types, the beneficial bacteria are no longer live and active. In such cases, the phrase "heat treated" must appear on the label.

To compensate for the weakness in the federal standards, in 1993, the National Yogurt Association (NYA) created the Live and Active Cultures (LAC) seal to be printed on the front display panel of yogurt containers, and the phrase "meets National Yogurt Association criteria for live and active culture yogurt" on the side display panel. The seal was devised to help dispel consumer confusion. In a consumer survey conducted by Opinion Research Corporation funded by NYA, nearly half of the respondents admitted that they did not know how to find out if a yogurt product contained live and active cultures. An overwhelming majority reported that it would be helpful to have a standard seal to identify yogurt products that contained live and active cultures.

In February 2000, NYA petitioned the FDA to amend the Standards of Identity for yogurt and to clarify the unclear existing standards. According to NYA, the standards were incomplete and provided consumers "little confidence" and manufacturers "little guidance as to how to properly meet them." The NYA proposed to identify yogurt as a food product that contains a minimum level of live and active cultures at the time of manufacture. According to the NYA, such an amendment would "boost consumer confidence by standardizing all yogurt products on the market." The petition included full-, low-, and non-fat types of yogurt with Standards of Identity. In addition, the NYA addressed issues such as acidity, homogenization/pasteurization, optional ingredients, and nomenclature.

Some members of Congress supported the NYA petition and urged the FDA to take action. Juanita Millender-McDonald (D-Calif) wrote to the agency that "the current standard is so vague it allows puddings and other products to be labeled as yogurt when they do not contain the health benefits of yogurt."

Six months after the petition had been submitted, Christine Lewis, director of the FDA's Office of Nutritional Products, Labeling, and Dietary Supplements, reported that the agency was unable to reach a decision due to "limited resources." Lewis continued: "However, we recognize the importance of reinventing food standards in a manner that both protects the interest of consumers and provides manufacturers reasonable flexibility in using innovative techniques to produce foods governed by a standard of identity."

Parse this statement carefully. The phrase "provides manufacturers reasonable flexibility in using innovative techniques" translates to a continuation of the lax policy to allow junk-food yogurts to be labeled yogurt. The FDA was established to protect trusting consumers against the wiles of the marketplace. The first FDA Commissioner, Harvey Washington Wiley, M.D., would have rejected any concession to manufacturers for reasonable flexibility that would lead to food adulteration and consumer deception.

Qualifying for the LAC Seal

Many, but not all, yogurt manufacturers signed on with the NYA to use the LAC seal. Companies such as Dannon, Yoplait, and Häagen Daz decided to use it. Separate seals were needed for each different type of yogurt product, such as whole-, low-, and non-fat milk yogurts and for aspartame-sweetened yogurts. Members of the NYA were not required to pay an application fee, at least not for the first several types of seals that were approved. Voting members received ten free types of seals; nonvoting members, five free types. Nonmembers were required to pay $2,500 per type.

Gary Hirshberg, president of Stonyfield Farm, a yogurt company in Londonderry, New Hampshire, decided not to apply for the seal, even though its product exceeded the NYA standard. According to Hirshberg, the seal might be just a "marketing tool" that could *create* rather than *relieve* confusion. Most refrigerated yogurt already contained at least the level of live and active cultures set by the NYA. As a result, products that met the standard but did not bear the seal might be viewed, unfairly, as inferior and therefore placed at a competitive disadvantage. (Similar problems had arisen with a "Heart Healthy" seal for other food products.)

For a company to qualify for the LAC seal, it needed to submit data from an independent laboratory showing that its product contained live and active cultures at a level of at least 10 million bacteria per gram. According to Kroger, mentioned earlier, 10 million bacteria actually is "a low number considering that yogurt can have up to 100 times that much."

No federal standards exist for frozen yogurt. Some states, notably California, New York, and New Jersey, require the presence of active, viable bacteria in the frozen product. However, the regulations fail to specify the amounts. Ordinary refrigerated yogurt contains hundreds of millions, even billions of live active bacteria. Frozen yogurt contains few.

Certified Laboratories in Corona, Queens, New York, analyzed samples of frozen yogurt at the request of the *New York Times*. The tests showed that there were 2.6 billion live active bacteria per gram in plain refrigerated yogurt. The closest that any frozen yogurt came was only 130 million bacteria per gram. The remainder of the frozen yogurts tested ranged from tens of millions to the low thousands. One frozen yogurt product was as low as 6,210 bacteria per gram.

YOGURT AS A FUNCTIONAL FOOD

Americans have long held a belief that all bacteria are bad. Fortunately, this belief is changing due to greater accessibility and recognition of yogurt, kefir, and other fermented milk products as beneficial.

Yogurt, with its many transformations, has been swept along in a relatively new concept of "functional foods." The term is applied to foods that offer special health benefits, often because something has been added. Development in this field could only open up after the FDA relaxed regulations and allowed food processors to make certain health claims for products. For example, it is permissible for a processor of orange juice to claim that the calcium added to the juice helps to maintain strong bones.

Shopping for a Good Yogurt Product

Shopping for a good yogurt product is like searching for the proverbial needle in the haystack. Among many of the products in the refrigerated cases, look for the following features of good yogurt. It should be plain, unflavored yogurt made from whole milk (full fat). The reason for this choice was discussed earlier. Look for the phrase "contains live and active cultures" on the container. If the phrase reads "made with live cultures" reject the product. The phrase is deceptive. Of course, the produce was *made* with live cultures, or the milk would not have been converted to yogurt. The phrase indicates that the product has been repasteurized and no longer contains live and active cultures. This tricky phrase should be prohibited.

Read the ingredient panel. It should list milk, the culturing bacteria, and any added bacteria such as *L. acidophilus, L. reuteri, L. bifidus,* or *L. casei* (all are good), but nothing else. Reject any product that lists thickeners or stabilizers, such as starches and/or gelatin.

Look for the "pull date" or phrase "best used by (date)" on the container. Compare the dates on the products at the front of the refrigerated case with the dates on the products in the back of the case. Stores rotate stock of perishable items, including yogurt and dairy products. The front of the case may have older products than in the back of the case. You may need to learn the skill of reaching and stretching! At home, use the yogurt within a reasonable amount of time. Over weeks, the yogurt may still be edible and safe, but there is a gradual decline in the activity of the beneficial bacteria for which yogurt is eaten. Discard any yogurt that develops mold.

Selecting plain, unflavored yogurt does not mean that you have to eat it plain. You can add fruits and berries at home, and avoid the jams, concentrated fruit juices, added colorings and flavorings, and high amounts of sweeteners.

To use a yogurt-containing creamy salad dressing, you need not purchase a costly and inferior commercial product. Simply blend plain yogurt with your usual choices of olive oil, vinegar or lemon juice, and herbs.

Yogurt is a good substitute for sour cream or buttermilk. If you purchase whole-milk (full-fat) yogurt, the rich butterfat may be at the top. You can use it as a substitute for crème fraîche.

Functional foods have become highly profitable for the food industry. By adding substances that cost pennies, or even a thousandth of a cent, processors can raise the prices of products substantially due to the perception of "added value." The benefits to the consumer are less clear. Using the example of the addition of calcium to orange juice, has it actually helped maintain strong bones? The approach is simplistic. Many nutrients, in addition to calcium, are needed to maintain strong bones. Also, not all forms of calcium are absorbed and utilized efficiently. Other factors, including weight-bearing exercise, are additional consideration.

Inevitably, yogurt products would be reinvented as functional foods. Yogurt might be regarded as the poster child. It was a functional food long before the concept was even conceived. Now, food processors are promoting yogurt, in its new transformation as a functional food, with embellishments of bells and whistles, and also with high price tags. Yet, it is questionable whether these new functional versions truly offer any advantage over plain yogurt with live and active cultures.

Probiotic-Fortified Yogurts

The trend that Niklas Bjärum, sales and marketing director of Probi, predicted is well on its way. The shift in American perception is attributable largely to the introduction in 2006 of Dannon's Activia. The product is comparable to Actimel, produced by Dannon's parent company, Danone, a major French dairy. The new product was successful in the United States. The headline of an article in the *New York Times* (Jan 12, 2007) proclaimed, "IN LIVE BACTERIA FOOD MAKERS SEE A BONANZA." In the article, Andrew Martin reported that Activia is a yogurt with special viable bacteria. Within the year, sales soared and reached well past $100 million. Very few newly introduced food products in America achieve such spectacular sales. On the contrary, their failure rate is exceedingly high. The success was so heady that in 2007, Dannon expanded its line of probiotic dairy products, and introduced DanActive and Danimals.

Activia was promoted heavily on television as well as in print. The health claim for the product is that it "helps naturally to regulate your digestive system in two weeks." Dannon reported that this claim was based on clinical studies.

Dannon had funded four studies. Healthy men and women consumed 4 to 12 ounces of Activia daily. After two weeks, on average, it required ten to thirty fewer hours of transit time for food to travel through the gastrointestinal (GI) tract. Reduced transit time can reduce gas and bloating in healthy individuals, according to Miguel Freitas, Dannon's scientific affairs manager. However, prior to the studies, the healthy participants chosen had not been suffering from any digestive distress, nor did they have any history of GI tract problems. The study did not measure gas output, nor were the participants even asked if they felt better at the end of the studies. Individuals who suffer chronically from GI tract problems were not selected for the studies (*Biosci Microflora*, 2001; *Alimentary Pharmacology and Therapeutics*, 2002; and *Microbial Ecology in Health and Disease*, 2003).

The ingredient listing on Activia labels shows that the product contains sweeteners and many of the other undesirable additives as those found in some other yogurt products. The probiotic contained in the product is *Bifidum regularis* (named by Dannon with a patented term, *B. animalis* DN-173 010). The cost of the product (in 2007) was $20 to $60 for a month's supply, for one to three 4-ounce containers to be consumed daily. Plain yogurt may offer similar benefits, and at lower cost.

In 2008, a class action suit against Dannon charged that the company employed "massive and substantial" unsubstantiated gut- and digestive-health statements about Activia to justify its price of up to 30 percent more than regular yogurt products. The plaintiffs charged that "Dannon's representations are false, misleading, and reasonably likely to deceive the public." Furthermore, the suit accused Dannon of ignoring its own negative scientific findings, and demanded that Dannon launch a corrective advertising campaign.

Probiotic-Fortified Yogurt Drinks

Another Dannon product, DanActive, a probiotic-cultured dairy drink, also has been promoted heavily. The health claim alleges that the product helps strengthen the body's natural defenses (that is, the immune system) despite a stressful lifestyle. Who, among Americans, does not have a stressful lifestyle?

For the DanActive drink, Dannon conducted only one study. In Italy, 180 men and women, averaging sixty-seven years of age, consumed two 3.5-ounce bottles—7 ounces total—of the drink daily for two weeks. Another 180 men and women were matched and served as the control. Results showed that the participants who drank DanActive were just as likely to have GI tract problems and colds as the untreated control group. The treated group suffered from their colds an average of one and a half days shorter in duration than the untreated group. During the study, one out of four in the treated group suffered from so much gas, bloating, and nausea that the researchers had to lower the daily allotment of the product by half (only one bottle) (*Journal of Nutrition, Health, and Aging,* 2003).

The probiotic bacteria in DanActive drink is *Lactobacillus casei immunitas* (named by Dannon with a patented term *L. casei* DN-114 001). The cost of the product (in 2007) was $40 a month for two bottles daily. The bottles contain 3.3 ounces; two bottles, totaling 6.6 ounces, is slightly less than the 7 ounces used originally in the study. If one were to use a probiotic dairy drink such as plain kefir, the substitution would be less costly, and perhaps be equally effective.

Danimals, another recently introduced product by Dannon, contains *L. acidophilus* GG. The product targets young children, with brightly colored animals printed on a six-pack container. The individual servings of 4.1 ounces have different flavors. The product contains the usual objectionable sweeteners and other additions. There is no reason to sell a specialized yogurt product for young children. It is a marketing ploy. The individual servings and packaging add considerable cost to such products.

It is difficult to compare prices for Dannon's probiotic-added yogurts because there are different versions and sizes of each product. The best way to compare prices is to note the unit prices per pound for each product. As of 2007 (before the price of milk products and other foods rose sharply), Activia sold for $2.40 per pound; DanActive, $3.09; and Danimals, $5.15. The unit price for a quart of Stonyfield Farm organic yogurt was $2.00 per pound. It is obvious that Danimals, the child-targeted yogurt, was *more than double* the price of a competitor.

Despite these recent introductions of yogurt products hailed as probiotics, Stonyfield Farm has added beneficial bacteria to its products for years, without any fanfare. In addition to the live cultures necessary to produce the yogurt, this company has chosen to add *L. acidophilus, L. bifidus, L. casei, L. reuteri,* and *L. rhamnosus.*

In a 2006 report, the American Society for Microbiology noted that "at present, the quality of probiotics available to consumers in food products around the world is unreliable." What is needed is a research project, conducted by independent scientists, comparing the benefits of these commercial probiotic-containing dairy products with plain whole-milk yogurt with live and active cultures. To my knowledge, this has not been done.

Probiotic-Fortified Spin-Offs

The first probiotic digestive wellness cereal is claimed for a grain product. Kashi Vive cereal is cultured with a patented *L. acidophilus* LA-14. The health claim made for the product is that it "promotes digestive balance and immunity." At present, there are no published studies to support the claim. The cost of the product is about $27 a month for a daily serving of one and one-fourth cupfuls. At nearly $1 a day for this product, it would be less costly, and perhaps just as beneficial, to eat a wholegrain cereal and plain yogurt (and not necessarily in combination).

Predictably, "probiotics" has become a buzzword. It is generating a niche market. The trend is illustrated by two recent introductions. Probiotic drops have been designed to be given to infants from birth onward, even though infants at birth have probiotics in their GI tracts. Also, probiotic chewing gums have been launched, that allegedly prevent tooth decay. No proof for the claim was offered, but it was stated that the chewing of gum prevents harmful bacteria from sticking to teeth and attacking them.

Globally, functional foods with yogurt are expanding. In 2007, in Canada, Kraft launched a probiotic-containing cheddar cheese, called Kraft LiveActive. The product will be introduced into the United States, too. The company reported that the product contains more than one million *Bifidobacterium lactis* and *Lactobacillus rhamnosus* cultures per serving. These probiotic bacteria, heat sensitive, would be reduced if the consumer uses such cheese in cooking.

A kefir product was introduced by Lifeway Foods as Cultured Milk Smoothie Yogurt. The company claims that the product contains "Ten Live and Active Kefir Cultures," including *Streptococcus florentinus, Leuconostoc lactis* subsp. *cremoris,* and *Bifidobacterium longum.*

Platinum in yogurt? In Japan, flecks of gold leaf in sake have been a time-honored practice when the beverage was given as a gift to signify best wishes for good fortune. Now, another metal is being added to a food. Nippon Luna, a Japanese yogurt and fermented beverage company, launched Platinum Yogurt that builds on the gold-in-sake tradition. Four nanograms of platinum colloid are added to each container of yogurt. This product was researched by Professor Yusei Miyamoto at Tokyo University. The Japanese government permits nanosize particles of platinum as a food additive. The platinum nanocolloids are 3.3 nanometers (billionths of a meter). They are thought to be unusually powerful as an antioxidant. The package of the yogurt has a metallic silver color to emphasize its platinum content, thought to appeal to consumers attracted to trendy products. The product is promoted with a phrase, roughly translated, "We will prevent you from getting rusty."

"Daily-dose yogurt shots are a convenient way to improve consumers' diets," reported *Prepared Foods* in April 2007. "In the Netherlands, Campina released a yogurt drink under the Campina Optimel Control brand. Prepared with skimmed yogurt and sweeteners, this functional dairy drink contains fractioned vegetable oil (made from natural plant extracts) that suppresses the appetite."

In Ireland, Glanbia Consumer Foods introduced Lose Weight Health Shots under the Yoplait Essence Lose Weight brand. The claim for this product is that it enhances weight loss in dieting regimens.

In Japan, Kirin (with its beer manufacturing expertise) and Yakult (with its well-known research on probiotic bacteria) combined forces to launch BBcube under the Kirin Well-Foods brand. According to *Prepared Foods* (Apr 2007), "these crispy cubes contain Yakult's bifidobacteria and Kirin's beer yeast dietary fiber, which supplement each other for healthy gut flora."

Flowers Foods launched Mrs. Freshley's Snack Away Peanut Butter Wafers with the claim on the front of the package "Contains Probiotics." The ingredient panel lists *L. rhamnosus*.

Attune Foods introduced Cool Mint Chocolate, a candy bar with a claim "Probiotics good for life!" The front panel of the package proclaims "more than 5X the live active cultures in yogurt" and "Keeps Your Body Humming." On the Attune website, the company claims that each bar contains "more than 10 billion probiotics" and that the bars are formulated to "ensure each bar contains an effective number of probiotics when purchased." The probiotics are a mix of *B. lactis*, *L. acidophilus*, and *L. paracasei*.

Exploitation of yogurt seems to be limited only by the imagination of food technologists. In 2002, *Food Technology* reported that "Germany's Ehrmann AG offers kids crackling yogurts with Pop Rocks in cola and bubble gum flavors." Whatever happened to plain-Jane yogurt?

YOGURT'S NEXT TRANSFORMATION?

In the article "The Dominant Culture: Yogurt for the Masses," Kimberly J. Decker, contributing editor of *Food Product Design*, predicted in the April

2001 issue that fortification with nutraceuticals and minerals will "pump up the nutritional merits of yogurt," and create "a fertile field for new product development." Decker provided some examples:

> "Soy isoflavone's health benefits have led some yogurt manufacturers to consider supplementing cow's milk formulas with soy. . . . Omega-3 fatty acids will eventually find a place in yogurt, along with coenzyme Q_{10}. Adding these fat-soluble nutraceuticals to low- or non-fat yogurt systems should require emulsifiers, such as polysorbate-80 for dispersal. The medicinal flavor of herbs and fishy aroma of fish oils also fade with the help of encapsulation systems. Yogurt and yogurt-beverage manufacturers are looking to fortify their products with minerals like calcium, magnesium, and selenium . . . these metallic-tasting substances, especially with a low pH that can encourage deleterious reactions or their propensity to encourage oxidative rancidity must be monitored. But encapsulation technologies—as well as the addition of antioxidants such as vitamins C and E—bode well for the future of nutritionally pumped-up yogurts."

Pumped-up yogurt, anyone?

CHAPTER 13

Drinkable Cultured Milk

Yogurt is spoonable. Many drinkable cultured milk products also exist. A few are sold in food stores, and others are available only as home-made beverages. Like yogurt, the drinkable ones contain live active probiotic bacteria that help maintain a healthy gastrointestinal (GI) tract.

ACIDOPHILUS MILK

The values of *Lactobacillus acidophilus* bacteria have been described earlier as beneficial probiotics that are implantable in the human intestine. Some dairies in the United States had produced acidophilus-containing milk before 1975.

In order to culture the milk, dairies had to heat it to a very high temperature over an extended period of time, prior to inoculating it with the lactobacilli. During the growth of the bacteria, a high degree of acidity developed. The finished product had a markedly cooked flavor and a strong tartness. As a result, acidophilus milk was unappealing to the American palate, and the product had limited sales. The product was purchased mainly by individuals with lactose intolerance or by persons who perceived it as a "health food."

Probiotics in Acidophilus Milk

As early as 1931, attempts were made to grow *L. acidophilus* in a sterile medium, harvest the cells, and add them to pasteurized milk to obtain a bacterial population comparable to that in regular acidophilus milk. The process resulted in an unfermented product that maintained a flavor similar to regular pasteurized milk. At temperatures from 2° to 5°C (roughly 90° to 100°F) it was possible to keep the milk sweet for as long as a week. The *L. acidophilus* cell count in the treated milk did not decrease as rapidly as in regular acidophilus milk with its low pH.

Feeding studies with humans demonstrated that the *L. acidophilus* bacteria in the unfermented milk were implantable in the human intestine. The proof was supplied by measuring the *L. acidophilus* in the fecal samples of the participants in the studies. However, the acidophilus milk was not commercialized.

In the years that followed, there were major developments in finding ways to preserve bacterial cells by drying, freeze-drying, and by storing them in a frozen state. In 1959, researchers were successful in using a frozen concentrate of *L. acidophilus* to prepare a palatable acidophilus milk. The concentrate contained a sufficient number of viable cells that could be added to a pint or quart of whole milk for consumption. Or, a portion of it could be added to a glass of milk, and the remainder saved to treat additional milk later. The researchers suggested that the distribution of frozen concentrate to consumers would provide the means to obtain acidophilus milk for therapeutic use in a palatable form. However, as with the earlier attempt, the product had limited marketability.

Subsequent developments benefited the frozen concentrated starter cultures. Liquid nitrogen, an inert substance, became available and useful for freezing substances. Also, processors learned how to manufacture large quantities of bacterial cells aseptically. This development reduced the former production costs of needing to propagate and develop starter cultures in milk-culturing processing plants.

By the late 1960s, research was begun that resulted in a quantum leap for acidophilus milk. Marvin L. Speck, who as the William Neal Reynolds Professor of Food Science and Microbiology at North Carolina State University in Raleigh, led a team that attempted to produce a palatable acidophilus milk. Their efforts were funded by the National Dairy Council (NDC). In 1975 after more than five years of research, the team announced that it had developed an acidophilus milk that would be acceptable to consumers. The product lacked the unappealing flavor, and its taste actually was indistinguishable from regular milk. Yet, the new product had all the beneficial effects of acidophilus present in the former product.

The team had selected a culture that had been isolated from a human intestine, and purified and tested it to ensure that it conformed to the characteristics of authentic *L. acidophilus*. Then they determined the cultural requirements to produce the cells in large volume, and for the cells to be able to thrive and grow in the presence of bile salts. (It was known that lactobacilli in human feces possess the ability to grow in the presence of bile salts. Lactobacilli that are not found in feces do not possess this culturing characteristic.)

The bacteria in the new acidophilus milk were programmed to remain inactive as long as the milk remained at a temperature below 75°F. When ingested, the body's heat activated the bacteria so that they could break down lactose for easier digestion. The product was unsuited for cooking or as an addition to hot beverages, because cooking destroyed the qualities of the bacteria added for special benefits.

The researchers completed two years of clinical trials with a number of families of faculty members at North Carolina State University who volunteered to consume the treated milk. The participants had been given a pasteurized milk to which a frozen concentrate of the *L. acidophilus* culture had been added. No flavor problems were reported. The lactobacilli were found to survive passage into the intestine. This finding was established by identifying an increased number of *L. acidophilus* bacteria in the feces of the participants during the feeding period, and that continued even for a short time after the trial had ended.

On the basis of the success of the clinical trials, in 1975, the NDC Foundation introduced the treated milk as "Sweet Acidophilus" milk, a trademarked product. The foundation made arrangements with G. P. Gundlach & Company of Cincinnati, Ohio, a merchandising and licensing entity, which in turn, enfranchised Crowley Foods of Syracuse, New York, to market the product. The foundation also had an agreement with Marshall Products, a division of Miles Laboratory at Elkhart, Indiana, to produce frozen concentrates of the culture. Gundlach chose to market the product with the trade name "Nu-Trish."

The new dairy product was hailed by dairy industry sources as the most significant development in dairying since 1944 when vitamin D was added to milk.

Health Benefits of Sweet Acidophilus Milk

In promoting Sweet Acidophilus milk, the researchers described the health benefits of the product. In a surprisingly frank manner, they denounced the shortcomings of food products developed by fellow food processors. William M. Roberts, head of the Department of Food Sciences at North Carolina State University and a colleague of Speck's, in an interview with the *Transylvania Times* (Brevard, North Carolina) said that many modern foods, especially snack foods, are highly processed and virtually sterile, containing few or no microorganisms. Roberts contin-ued, "A diet of sterile foods tends to make the consumer more susceptible to disorders of the gastrointestinal tract. We need to put more emphasis on the types of foods that help maintain a healthy balance of microorganisms in the gastrointestinal tract."

Speck agreed with Roberts and noted that in the past, when people ate more raw foods, they had more lactobacilli naturally. That situation no longer holds, with today's highly processed foods.

In a leaflet printed by Idlewild, a New England dairy, mention was made that intestinal balance was important because "today in America our diets tend to result in a deficiency of the needed *L. acidophilus* bacteria due to the extensive consumption of sterile foods and the use of food preservatives."

Materials supplied to dairies by the NDC were used on the side panels of cartons containing acidophilus milk. The text on cartons of the product from Muller-Pinehurst Dairy serving northern Illinois, read in part that "*L. acidophilus* culture is a scientific name of a strain of beneficial bacteria which scientific literature reports may be lacking in our digestive systems because of the manner in which present-day foods are refined, sterilized, and preserved."

Although the acidophilus milk clearly had benefits, there were federal roadblocks that prevented any health claims from being made for a food in interstate commerce. The NDC requested information from the Food and Drug Administration (FDA) as to what could be stated on labels. The NDC was referred to the compliance division. According to the NDC's account, related to dairy companies:

> We were told "You can't do it" to every suggestion we made about what we wanted to say about the benefits of the product. We wound up with this about the policy: you can do analytical—or what we would call compositional analysis for labeling; you can say you've got a certain percentage of this in your product, going from protein right on down, or you can express it as a percentage of your needs in one serving, and this sort of thing. But if you make any health claim, such as the calcium in milk is good for you, or the protein in milk is good for you, you'll be sent over to the Food and Drug Division. How can dairy industry people go about nutrition education if you can't say anything about the health benefits of your product?

Nevertheless, distribution of Sweet Acidophilus milk went national. Wherever the product was introduced, sales were stymied by the FDA's insistence that no health claim could be made. Rolf Thienemann, vice president and sales manager of the Muller-Pinehurst Dairy, asserted that "It is difficult for people to understand what Sweet Acidophilus milk is, if you cannot make any specific claim about it."

Maverick dairies that promoted the product with health claims were lassoed promptly. For example, Russell Farms in Great Neck, New York, was forced to drop its claim that Sweet Acidophilus milk helps digestion and prevents systemic intestinal infections for healthy consumers. The claims were truthful and supportable by scientific data. Yet New York State Attorney General Louis J. Lefkowitz took action. Without conceding any wrongdoing, Russell Farms agreed to cease making claims and paid a $3,000 fine. The claims were accurate, supportable, and modest. Currently, with the FDA's approval for certain health claims, many are inaccurate, unsupportable, and misleading. Yet, they are tolerated.

In an attempt to inform the public, dairies held press conferences for the media, at which consultants such as dietitians from schools, hospitals, nursing homes, and other institutions, spoke favorably about the new product. Local news media recognized the new product as one of interest, and afforded it substantial space in print media, and in time on radio and television newscasts. Gradually, the new product achieved widespread recognition and distribution. The treated milk cost only pennies more than regular milk. The product was well received by consumers.

In recent times, however, other introductions have superseded the product. Lactaid, a commercial product that can be added to milk, reduces the lactose, and makes the milk better tolerated by individuals with lactose intolerance. The product has been used by some dairies to produce treated milk. Lactaid is available, too, in stores so that consumers can add the product at home to regular milk. Also, the development of probiotic dietary supplements, discussed in Appendix A on page 153, has impacted strongly on the declined sale and consumption of acidophilus milk.

KEFIR

Kefir originated centuries ago in the Caucasus Mountains of Russia. It was customary to prepare kefir by pouring soured milk into leather bags known as *burdiuki.* Over time, some of the kefir culture that adhered to the walls of the bag was collected, air-dried, and stored for later use. It would be reconstituted in fresh milk. Kefir was known as *kunney* by the Mongols, inhabitants of the Russian steppes, the Kalmuks, the Kirghiz, and other groups of people. The kefir, carried in the burdiuki, accompanied these groups during long caravan journeys.

Today, we still enjoy kefir, either the commercial product, or the homemade one. Commercial kefir was available in some areas since 1945. Now, it is available nationally, and is found in refrigerated cases in grocery stores in proximity to fresh milk. For people who wish to make kefir at home, there are two possible sources of the culturing substance. Either it can be purchased in freeze-dried form and reconstituted, or it may be shared by someone whose culturing substance has grown to such an extent that it can be divided.

Unflavored kefir is similar in flavor and texture to good quality buttermilk. Actually, it has been used by some dairies to produce "cultured" buttermilk. Kefir's texture is thicker than fluid milk but thinner than yogurt.

Kefir's Nutritional and Therapeutic Values

All cultured milks share some commonality, but have some unique characteristics. Kefir has many of the same nutritional and therapeutic values of other cultured milks. Based on various studies, kefir, like other cultured milks, has demonstrated properties that benefit the GI tract and immune system, inhibit tumor formation, and lower cholesterol.

Kefir also has some unique features. It has very low-curd tension, so the curd readily breaks up into extremely small particles (unlike yogurt's curds that hold together or separate into clumps). The small particle-size curds help its digestion by presenting a large surface for the digestive agents to utilize. For this reason, kefir has been recommended as an ideal food for infants, convalescents, the elderly, and individuals with impaired digestive activity. Also, it has been found that kefir stimulates saliva flow probably due to its acidity and slight carbonation. It increases the flow of digestive juices and stimulates peristalsis in the GI tract. This feature has made kefir useful as a postoperative food after abdominal operations that can cause temporary cessation of peristalsis and the resulting gas pains. Sigurd Orla-Jensen, a noted Danish dairy bacteriologist, recommended kefir over yogurt because he thought that kefir had a higher nutritive value due to the abundance of digestible yeast cells that benefit intestinal flora.

Kefir, like yogurt, contains less lactose than regular milk. Is kefir, like yogurt, useful for lactose intolerant individuals? To answer this question, Steven R. Hertzler and Shannon M. Clancy, both at the medical dietetic division of the School of Allied Medical Professions, Ohio State University in Columbus, selected fifteen adults who were healthy but were lactose intolerant. The researchers divided the participants into three groups. Each group was fed test meals, and also given milk, kefir, or yogurt. Both the kefir and yogurt-consuming groups had similar reduced severity of flatulence by 54 to 71 percent relative to the milk-consuming group (the control). Abdominal pain and diarrheal symptoms, common for lactose intolerant individuals who attempt to drink milk, were negligible for the yogurt and kefir groups. The researchers suggested that kefir improved lactose digestion and tolerance, and might be a helpful strategy in coping with lactose intolerance.

Probiotics in Kefir

The starter for culturing kefir is known as kefir "grains." They are not cereal based, but in appearance, are small, hard, yellow-white, irregularly shaped granules that clump together and resemble miniature cauliflower heads. The grains consist of masses of bacteria, lactose-fermented yeasts, polysaccharides (multiple sugars), and other products of bacterial metabolism, along with the curds of insoluble milk casein (a protein). The bacteria and yeasts work well in tandem.

The species of bacteria and yeasts in the kefir grains may vary, depending on the geographic location. Typically, kefir starter culture has a larger and more diverse range of microorganisms than does yogurt. For example, the culture used by Lifeway Foods in Morton Grove, Illinois, the largest kefir producer in the country, contains *Streptococcus lactis*, *Lactobacillus plantarum*, *Streptocccoccus cremoris*, *Lactobacillus casei*, *Streptococcus diacetylactis*, *Saccharomyces florentinus*, and *Leuconostoc cremoris*. Lifeway Foods also adds a concentrated bovine colostrum to some of its kefir products. (See Appendix C on Colostrum on page 169.)

Kefir is produced by adding the kefir grains to fresh milk, and allowing it to remain at room temperature from twelve hours up to a few days, depending on the degree of desired tartness. Then the granules are strained out of the cultured kefir and transferred to a new batch of fresh milk. If the kefir is made at home, no special equipment is needed. The culture can be kept alive and active for years, without having to be discarded and replaced. A thriving culture will multiply, in which case, it can be divided and shared. Or, it can be dried, and stored for future use, at which time it is reconstituted by soaking the granules in fresh milk. Or, the culture can be frozen by placing the grains in a small dark glass bottle, capped tightly, and stored in a freezer. The dark glass protects the culture from light, and the tight capping protects the culture from oxygen. Both light and oxygen are destructive. The frozen kefir grains are in a quiescent state, and can be revived and activated after being defrosted.

The dual fermentation by the lactic acid bacteria and the yeasts results in a small amount of carbon dioxide being formed. It produces a mild carbonation in the kefir. Also, a low level (0.01 to 0.10 grams per 100 grams) of alcohol is produced. The combination of carbonation and alcohol has earned kefir a reputation as "the champagne of milk."

BUTTERMILK

Modern commercial buttermilk has little in common with traditional buttermilk, and nothing to do with modern butter production. Traditional buttermilk, simply termed "buttermilk" is unavailable. "Cultured buttermilk" is the product sold in stores, in proximity to cartons of fluid milk.

Real buttermilk was a byproduct of farm-made butter. During the churning, when butter began to form from the cream, the liquid was drained off through a hole in the bottom of the churn. During the churning process the liquid became slightly sour from airborne bacteria. The liquid had flecks of butter from the churning. Unless the liquid was strained, the flecks of butter remained in the liquid and gave it a buttery flavor. This slightly soured liquid was buttermilk. Being unpasteurized, the liquid contained the lactic acid-producing bacteria that allowed the liquid to ferment and produce buttermilk. The acid prevented pathogenic microorganisms from spoiling the product during its fermentation.

With the growth of creameries, butter production was transferred from the farm to the dairy company. Arthur Jensen Een, a dairyman who grew up in a community settled by Scandinavians in central Wisconsin, recalled his experience in the 1920s. His mother would send him to the cooperative creamery where he could purchase a gallon of buttermilk for one cent! At the time, buttermilk was regarded as a waste product. Most of it was poured into tanks, hauled away, and added to hog feed. A small amount was kept for a few customers willing to pay for the waste product. Een viewed current buttermilk as "a sort of cultured imitation."

Probiotics in Buttermilk

Presently sold cultured buttermilk, as noted earlier, has nothing to do with butter production. The process is similar to that of making yogurt. The dairy starts with pasteurized skim milk to which pasteurized non-fat milk solids may be added. Because the milk lacks live acid-producing bacteria, it cannot ferment properly. The milk is inoculated with bacteria, usually *S. lactis*. Because the milk is not actually in contact with any butter, a buttery flavor must be supplied. At times, flecks of butter have been added to simulate old-time buttermilk. More frequently, *Leuconostoc citrovorum* is added. This bacterium converts a small amount of citric acid into diacetyl, a volatile molecule with a butterlike flavor.

The incubation period for cultured buttermilk is about twelve hours, at a low temperature of about 70°F. This is the best temperature for diacetyl production. The incubation period for cultured buttermilk is longer than for yogurt, and the temperature is lower than for yogurt. Stabilizers may be added to the product in order to increase viscosity in the product.

The quality of commercial cultured buttermilk may vary. Researchers at the University of Georgia examined eight brands of cultured buttermilk from local retail outlets. The researchers analyzed the products on the day of purchase. All brands showed high pathogenic counts. Of the eight brands tested, seven were contaminated with coliform bacteria. There were large variations in the concentration of diacetyl, acetoin, and acetaldehyde. Acetaldehyde is responsible for a flavor defect, sometimes found in cultured buttermilk, and termed "green apple." Of the eight brands tested, 73 percent were rated only fair to poor.

Like yogurt, buttermilk has undergone a transformation. Starting as a waste product, it has become a product of commerce. Consumers should regard cultured buttermilk as a product of less worth than that of a good-quality kefir or acidophilus milk. However, on a positive note, cultured buttermilk does offer nutrients, and would be a far better choice than a soft drink. Also, cultured buttermilk is tolerated by lactose-intolerant individuals.

PIIMÄ

Piimä is a less-known cultured milk drink. To date, it is a product that is unavailable commercially. However, a commercial starter is available for making homemade piimä.

Piimä originated in Finland. In northern Europe, a wild herb, butterwort (genus *Pinguicola*) grows commonly in moist areas. It is a carnivorous plant. A rosette of leaves forms around its base. The leaves are coated with a sticky secretion that traps insects.

It was discovered that during the period of peak butterwort growth, cows grazing on this herb produced milk that clabbered (curdled) at room temperature. People used the clabbered milk as a starter to culture milk. A small amount of the cultured milk would be reserved from each batch to inoculate the subsequent batch. The cultured milk became known as piimä. The product has a custard-like texture. If handled roughly, by shaking or stirring, it separates.

The commercial freeze-dried starter must be refrigerated until it is used. The process of making piimä is very simple. The milk is placed in a clean container and the starter is added. The container is stored at room temperature in a cupboard or on a countertop. It should be covered to exclude light, and unwanted bacteria and wild yeasts present in the air. The ideal culturing temperature is between 72° and 75°F. If cooler, the culturing process will require more time; if warmer, the end product will be tarter. Depending on the temperature, piimä is cultured within eight to twenty-four hours. It will be slightly thick. After refrigeration for six to twelve hours, it will have thickened more, and is ready to eat. A small amount should be reserved in the refrigerator for culturing the subsequent batch.

Piimä has similar characteristics of other cultured milk products, but has a special feature. Other cultured milk products need to be heated to kill pathogens that would compete with the inoculated bacteria. Piimä requires no heating. This feature is attractive for individuals who favor drinking raw milk.

TAETTE

Taette is one of those numerous cultured milks commonly made at home, and currently unavailable commercially. Sometimes the culture is available from individuals, having been handed down from immigrants and carefully nurtured from generation to generation, and shared generously with others.

Taette originated in Norway. Farmwomen gathered some unspecified meadow plant with blue petals. They placed a few of the plant's leaves in bowls, poured boiled milk over the leaves, and set the bowls in warm cupboards or on windowsills in summertime. The milk thickened to a soft custard-like texture. After removing the leaves, the taette was eaten. A small amount was reserved to culture the next batch.

When milk was plentiful, taette was stored in casks or barrels. Great care was taken to spoon it out gently, because taette easily separates into curds and whey. Sometimes, taette was spooned into bowls and sour cream was added. It has been reported that the culturing leaves possessed such strong bioactivity that spring milk, converted to taette, would still be safe to drink by wintertime. By then, the taste and characteristics of the milk had changed, but it was still consumable.

When Norwegians emigrated they were reluctant to abandon their taette cultures. Doubtless, there were many experiments to find some way to transport the culture to a new location. One successful method was to dip a clean piece of linen into the taette and airdry it. Later, in the new location, the taette was reconstituted and found to be viable.

For me, this feat is a metaphor. Just as the emigrants faced an unknown future, so was the dormant culture facing an unknown future. Would either survive? Also, cultural ties are strong, and are especially strong for food traditions. By transplanting taette successfully, the emigrants retained their cultural heritage. The old and the new were connected. The past could be savored in the present, and there was hope that it could be savored in the future, as a vibrant milk-culturing agent would be passed along, from one generation to another.

OTHER DRINKABLE CULTURED MILKS

Numerous other traditional drinkable cultured milks have been enjoyed, as mentioned earlier in Chapter 3, "Fermneted Foods and Beverages Around the Globe." They deserve brief mention.

Skyr, a curdled milk, was common in Scandinavia. The milk was kept for months to make skyr. It was described as resembling milk "freshly drawn from the cow" but tasting like "vinegar mixed with something bitterer than aloe." Indeed, the Scandinavians used skyr as a vinegar substitute.

Scandinavians made *ymer* by inoculating milk with an acidifying bacterial culture. The mixture was allowed to sour, and then was heated to coagulate the proteins. The watery whey was pressed out, and the solids cooled. Cream and brown sugar were added, and the soft custard, ymer, was enjoyed for breakfast.

Kumiss originated among the nomadic Mongols in the Caucasus

Mountains. It was known as kumiss when made from mare's milk; *kephir*, from camel's milk; and *airan*, from yak's milk. Currently, it is made from cow's milk. Kumiss spread out from the Caucasus region. The Tartars called it *kumys, katky,* or *koumiss.* Inhabitants of the Russian steppes, the Mongolians, and others called it *kunney;* the Romanians, *kumys;* the Montenegrins, *kisla verenyka;* and in the Balkans, *kisselo mleko.*

The Mongols poured the milk into large leather pouches and allowed it to ferment. The liquid was beaten with a wooden stick to churn it. The beatings were done sporadically for several days to produce kumiss. In modern times, kumiss is still produced and drunk, especially by the Kazak people in Turkestan.

Kisk is a bacterially fermented product made from milk and parboiled wheat. It is fermented by lactic acid from the addition of yogurt as a starter. Kisk is a staple in the Middle East. In laboratory analysis, after fermentation, there is a slight rise in a vitamin B fraction, riboflavin. However, kisk is sometimes sun-dried. By doing this, the riboflavin, which is light sensitive, decreases.

The main fresh fermented milk product in Egypt is *zabady.* Minor ones are *laban rayeb, laban khad, laban zeer,* and *kishk* (kisk).

SOME SPREADABLE CULTURED MILK PRODUCTS

Some cultured milk products can be made into spreadable cheeses by draining the whey from the curds. A few of them are in commercial production, along with the vast array of popular fresh and aged cheeses.

Quark (also *qvark* or *quarg*) is a soft creamy unripened acid-cured spreadable cheese made from whole milk. It is native to Germany and France. Its use in the United States, to date, has been limited to its inclusion in the astronauts' meal program in a project at the Houston Space Center in Texas.

Bakers' cheese, related to quark, has some institutional use. Pot cheese, a ripened quark rind, is in limited commercial production.

Kurish is a fresh lactic acid cheese that is popular in Egypt.

Yogurt cheese, also known as *labneh,* is easy to make at home. Surprisingly, to my knowledge, it has never been developed as a commercial product. (To learn how to make your own, see the inset on the next page.)

SOURED CREAMS

Traditionally, soured creams such as clotted or clabbered products were made simply by allowing fresh cream to ferment by bacteria in the air when the cream was cultured in a shallow dish and set in a warm place. Devonshire cream was made from whole milk, heated slowly below the boiling point. The cream rose to the top and thickened. When the milk cooled, the cream was skimmed off the top.

The traditional method of making soured creams relied on lactic acid bacterial fermentation. Current sour cream products are processed quite differently, with a sped-up process that does not depend on fermentation.

Currently, commercial sour creams are made without any bacterial inoculation. Instead, an acidic medium, such as vinegar, is added to the cream to curdle the mixture. The product may not even contain cream. It

Homemade Yogurt Cheese

Line a colander with cheesecloth and set the colander over a deep pot or large bowl. Pour unflavored whole-milk yogurt into the colander, cover with a clean dishtowel, and allow the whey to drip overnight at room temperature. In the morning, carefully gather together the corners of the cheesecloth and tie them with a clean strong cord. Remove the colander and suspend the hanging cheesecloth over the pot or bowl by means of a dowel, and allow additional whey to drip through. *Do not squeeze the cheesecloth.* After the whey stops dripping, carefully empty the contents of the cheesecloth into a container with a cover. This is yogurt cheese, which tastes like a fine cream cheese of yesteryears, but alas, no longer is produced. Refrigerate the yogurt cheese and plan to use it within a few days.

You will find that a large amount of whey has separated from the curd (the cheese). You can drink it, add it to soups, stews, vegetable juices, or to the liquid in bread dough. Or, refrigerate it in a tightly closed glass jar for future use. The refrigerated whey will keep for several months. It makes an excellent starter for culturing vegetables, which will be discussed in Chapter 14. Or, if you cook a wholegrain cereal, soak the grains overnight at room temperature in water and add one or two teaspoonfuls of whey, or a teaspoonful of plain powdered whey sold in health food stores. The whey adds nutrients, but more importantly, it improves the digestibility of the cereal.

—Adapted from *A Whole Foods Primer,* Beatrice Trum Hunter (Basic Health Publications, 2007)

may be made from milk to which a number of additives achieve the texture and some resemblance to the taste and flavor of cultured sour cream.

In the late 1970s, an independent researcher-inventor brought an idea to the Battelle Development Corporation (BDC), a nonprofit subsidiary of the Battelle Memorial Institute in Columbus, Ohio.

The BDC is involved mainly in transferring or developing technology from the concept stage to commercial reality.

The inventor's idea, finally developed, made sour cream by a rapid, direct acidification method, rather than by bacterial action. The new process greatly reduced production time, and allowed for quality control of the texture, flavor, and acidity of the product. Because of the low bacterial count, the process extended the shelflife of the product.

The famous French crème fraîche, valued by cooks everywhere, is not made from fresh cream, but from mature (that is, fermented) cream. The naturally present lactic acid bacteria culture the cream, and make it thick with a distinctly agreeable flavor. Cooks like to use crème fraîche for these qualities, as well as for its ability not to curdle when heated. The genuine crème fraîche from France is made from heavy cream with a high-butterfat content (about 40 percent). Domestic crème fraîche, commercially available, has a lower butterfat content (about 30 to 36 percent). Discriminating cooks recognize the differences between the superior imported product and the domestically produced one. Madeleine Kamman, author of *When French Women Cook: A Gastronomic Memoir* (Ten Speed Press, 1976) cautioned American cooks that:

> Trying to make crème fraîche is a ridiculous waste of time, since the taste you are dreaming of comes from the combination of grass from meadows 4,000 miles over the ocean, milk from breeds of cows that do not exist in the United States, and bacterial fermentations that cannot be the same in the United States as they are in France.

For cooks who wish to achieve results that are somewhat like those by using crème fraîche, it is not necessary to purchase a pricey import. Nor is it necessary to slave in the kitchen, attempting to make crème fraîche. An excellent substitute is the cream at the top of a good-quality, unflavored whole-milk yogurt. As Thoreau advised, "Simplify, simplify."

PART THREE

Fermented Non-Dairy Foods

CHAPTER 14

Fermented Vegetables: Nutritional and Therapeutic Treasures

For many Americans, the most familiar fermented vegetable is sauerkraut. For Germans, it is the national dish. Like yogurt and other cultured milk products, fermented vegetables are products resulting from the action of lactic acid bacteria. Sometimes, the process is called lacto-fermentation, referring to the lactic acid. Or, such products may be termed cultured vegetables. Whatever the term, all fermented vegetables contribute nutrients, digestibility, and healthful qualities to the diet. They differ from yogurt and other cultured milk products insofar as they do not require inoculation with a bacterium to ferment them. Rather, fermented vegetables depend on free and wild unpatented bacteria present in the air.

PROBIOTICS IN FERMENTED VEGETABLES

Numerous health benefits are ascribed to fermented vegetables due to the lactic acid that cultures them. They are reported to

- stimulate the immune system

- contribute to protecting the body against infections

- improve the digestive process by regulating the acidity in the digestive tract and by stimulating beneficial intestinal flora production

- facilitate the synthesis of certain vitamins such as vitamin B_{12}, which can be produced only in the presence of lactic acid bacteria

- facilitate the breakdown and assimilation of proteins by means of the lactic acid and enzymes present in lacto-fermented vegetables

- benefit diabetics because the lactic acid bacteria convert the sugar content in the vegetable into a more assimilable component

• help prevent arthritis because the lactic acid does not have the harmful acidifying effect on the human system shown by other organic acids

• benefit the nervous system by having a soothing effect

• benefit individuals who have candidal infections and are eating a yeast-free diet

SAUERKRAUT

According to legend, the technique for making sauerkraut was used in ancient China, and sauerkraut was a staple food for the workers who constructed the Great Wall of China. The technique reached Europe from China via the Tartars.

In Europe, the elite regarded cabbage as an unsophisticated food that produced a foul odor when it was cooked, and flatulence when eaten. The peasantry, particularly in northern Europe, valued cabbage, especially when converted into sauerkraut. An abundant harvest crop of cabbages could be turned into a form that would preserve it for use during the long winter. Sauerkraut retains the vitamin C present in cabbage. The vitamin C protected the peasants against scurvy during the winter months when fresh berries and fruits were unavailable.

The northern Europeans brought their sauerkraut-making technique to the New World, and homemade sauerkraut was part of the activity of autumnal "putting by" as part of American farm life. By the 1940s, however, our food supply became radically changed. Many highly processed foods produced in factories were afforded long shelflife due to the use of several thousand chemical additives, some of dubious safety, added to the products. Basic home preparation of foods declined as more and more factory-produced foods were introduced. As more women entered the workplace, "built-in-maid service" of convenient foods became attractive.

Prior to the 1940s, basic cookbooks included instructions for making homemade sauerkraut and pickles. Printed instructions for making these fermented foods were readily available from the U.S. Department of Agriculture's (USDA) home economists and its agricultural extension service. After that period, it became rare to find such instructions in basic cookbooks, or from the USDA.

By then, commercially canned sauerkraut was available. It contained a very high salt level and a chemical preservative. These products bear little resemblance to raw lacto-fermented sauerkraut. The heat processing of the canned product results in some destruction of vitamin C. There is further depletion of the vitamin in long storage of the canned product, especially if it is stored in a warm place. The salt level is so high that it is necessary to rinse the sauerkraut in cold water to rid it of the excessive salt before it is consumed, even if the individual is not restricted to a low-sodium diet. The rinsing, itself, further depletes the sauerkraut of vitamin C, which is a water-soluble vitamin. Nor does canned sauerkraut bear any resemblance in flavor to its raw lacto-fermented counterpart.

Although supermarkets offer tens of thousands of food products, they rarely stock lacto-fermented sauerkraut or other lacto-fermented vegetables. Outlets such as health food stores usually stock refrigerated vacuum-packed lacto-fermented vegetables. The major brand is Bio Lacto/Deep Root Organic Raw Cultured Vegetables, produced by Caldwell Bio Fermentation Canada in Martinville, Quebec (www.biolacto.com).

Some people might wish to make homemade sauerkraut but are discouraged by the thought that the process involves the use of dozens of cabbages. No so. Sauerkraut can be made from a single head of cabbage, and easily stored even in a compact urban kitchen.

One of the few current cookbooks that offer instructions for making sauerkraut and other fermented foods is *Nourishing Traditions* by Sally Fallon with Mary G. Enig (New Trends Publishing, 1999).

Stated simply, lactic acid fermentation of a mixture of shredded cabbage and salt forms sauerkraut. The cabbage can be green or red. The salt can be added at a very low level (about one tablespoon of salt with four tablespoons of liquid whey, or two tablespoons of salt, without whey, for each head of cabbage) so that it is not necessary to rinse away the salt after homemade sauerkraut is completed.

The salt pulls the liquid out of the cabbage and helps prevent undesirable bacteria from growing. But the beneficial lactic acid-producing bacteria can still grow in the naturally occurring sugars present in the cabbage. They convert these sugars into acids, which give sauerkraut its agreeable tartness.

The beneficial bacteria work faster at warm temperatures, and slower at cooler ones. The cooler temperatures permit the bacteria to convert the sugars into acids slowly, and make the end product palatable.

Sauerkraut, like cabbage, is recognized as a good dietary source for vitamin C. During the period of active fermentation, the vitamin C level equals that of the original cabbage. This feature is surprising, because vitamin C (ascorbic acid) is lost readily. After fermentation is completed, there is a gradual decline in vitamin C, similar to the decline in long-stored cabbage.

A Great Cosmic Mystery

Tom Cowan, a San Francisco physician who is interested in traditional foods for natural healing, refers to lacto-fermented foods as "one of the great cosmic mysteries" for "there is a family of microorganisms that live on and around food, that when given a chance to flourish, turn ordinary foods . . . into rich nutritional and therapeutic treasures."

Cowan points out that although raw cabbage is a valuable and nourishing food, it can create problems (gas, goiter, hypothyroidism, and thyroid enlargement). Cooked cabbage loses some vitamin C. "Now comes the magic," says Cowan. "By some quirk of nature, or perhaps really it is by the wisdom of nature, on all cabbage leaves live certain bacteria, which, when provided with an anaerobic environment . . . accomplished by the simple addition of salt to the cabbage, begin to grow and thrive. They especially thrive when the cabbage leaves have been pulverized a bit (that is, shredded and pounded). And what magic they then do! First, they break down the substances that cause the goiter and the gas. Then, they produce . . . lactic acid, which 'cleanses' the bowels, and adds lactic acid bacteria, which have been widely [recognized] as immune stimulants and digestive aids. Then, to top it all off, another byproduct of the metabolism of these bacteria is the substance, acetylcholine, which is known to be a relaxing, calming tonic for the nervous system. Truly an alchemical magic act, to become healthful sauerkraut from such humble players—cabbage, salt, and bacteria."

Cabbage is in the Brassica family, along with brussels sprouts, cauliflower, and mustard greens. All of these vegetables have shown anticancer activity. Does sauerkraut have anticancer activity? Fermented cabbage has been found to block the action of estrogen, a hormone that can fuel the growth of breast cancer and other reproductive malignancies.

William G. Helferich, a nutritionist, headed a team at the University of Illinois at Urbana-Champagne, to answer this question. Immigrant Polish women have been found to be at far higher risk of developing breast cancer than their counterparts in Poland. One distinguishing factor is that the women in Poland consume far greater amounts of fermented cabbage than the women who have immigrated to America.

Helferich and his team set up a test tube experiment. They stimulated colonies of human breast cancer cells with estrogen. Then, they added low concentrations (5 to 25 parts per billion) of extracts of plain cabbage, sauerkraut, or acidified brussels sprouts. The extracts slowed the growth of estrogen-fed cells and also blocked the estrogen's ability to activate a particular gene associated with carcinogenesis. At parts per billion (ppb), the different potencies of the three vegetable preparations showed little difference in activity. However, at higher concentrations in parts per million (ppm), each extract mimicked estrogen. They stimulated cell growth and gene activity.

Helferich reported that "though it's very unlikely you'll get these higher concentrations in the blood from eating brassicas, it is realistic [that] you could get the antiestrogenic doses" (*Journal of Agricultural and Food Chemistry*, 2000).

PICKLES

Lacto-fermented cucumbers result in the old-fashioned pickles of my childhood. They were sold commonly from large open barrels in the immigrant neighborhoods of the lower East Side of Manhattan in the early 1900s. The cucumbers were submerged in a brine consisting solely of water and salt. The solution had enough salt to prevent the growth of undesirable microbes, but was weak enough to allow the growth and predominance of bacterial species that produce lactic acid. Often, such pickles were delicately flavored with sprigs of dill, cloves of garlic, bay leaves, and peppercorns. The pickles maintained their crispness without any chemical firming agent. Nor did they require any chemical preservative, other than the salt. The pickles tasted only mildly salty.

Such lacto-fermented cucumber pickles are distinctly different from most pickles currently sold. These cucumbers are cooked to a soft consistency or submerged briefly in brine to draw out moisture that otherwise would dilute the vinegar. Then, the cucumbers are submerged in the vinegar brine. Often, spices and sugar or sweeteners are added. Bacteria in the vinegar are almost entirely inactive, but molds and yeasts are still able to grow at a low pH and can contaminate the surface if it is uncovered. A preservative may be added to discourage contamination. Such pickled cucumbers are packed into jars, covered with brine, capped, and pasteurized. This method of brine preservation of pickles leads to a large loss or destruction of most of the nutrients present originally in the cucumbers. The water-soluble constituents are leached out into the vinegar brine and are largely discarded in a desalting operation prior to packing into jars. The sugars are fermented mostly to carbon dioxide and acids. In studies, such pickles lost 100 percent of their vitamin C, and from 75 to 85 percent of their vitamin B complex. For some puzzling and unexplained reason, the beta-carotene content was higher in the pickles than in the fresh cucumbers, but not high enough to be of nutritional significance. The role of such pickles is their contribution of variety and zest to the diet rather than nutrients, whereas the lacto-fermented pickles have health-promoting features similar to those of other fermented foods.

As with sauerkraut, directions for making lacto-fermented cucumber pickles were given commonly in early cookbooks, but dropped in more recent ones. Directions are included in *Wild Fermentation* by Sandor Ellix Katz (Chelsea Green, 2003).

It is difficult to find lacto-fermented cucumber pickles as well as good sauerkrauts in supermarkets. There are a few specialty stores that still sell pickles from barrels. Also, they are available in healthfood stores in refrigerated cases. They are packed in glass jars. One product is Real Pickles, produced in Montague, Massachusetts (www.realpickles.com).

KIMCHI

Kimchi (also spelled kimchee) is a Korean version of fermented cabbage. Its basic ingredients are cabbage, and other vegetables such as spring onions, flavored with garlic, ginger, and hot chili pepper.

Kimchi has had a long history of use in Korea. Its first mention was by an eminent Korean poet, Lee Kyu-bo (1168–1241). In the fifteenth century, the chili pepper was introduced from the New World into Europe. Ultimately, it found its way into the Far East. The introduction of the chili pepper into Korea resulted in traditional kimchi undergoing substantial changes.

The tradition continues. Fermented vegetables have long been vital in the Korean diet during the long, harsh winters, a time when fresh vegetables are unavailable. Kimchi is reported to retain the nutrients of fresh vegetables quite well after the vegetables are fermented.

Space-Age Kimchi?

With its venerable history of use, kimchi may be launched into the space age. Scientists at the Korea Atomic Energy Research Institute in Daejeon announced in 2006 that they processed a special kimchi to launch with Korea's first astronaut to join the Russian spaceship, *Soyuz.*

Working with researchers at the Institute of Biomedical Problems, a Russian government facility that conducts biomedical support for space flights, Myung Woo Byun, a Korean scientist, led a team in developing a system to make kimchi practical as a space travel food. The team subjected fully fermented kimchi to gamma and electro-irradiation to sterilize the food. Then, they froze it to a semi-dried state, and packed it into a vacuum-sealed pouch.

"Space food is now entirely Western food, so we thought it would be meaningful to have a Korean food on the menu," reported Byun. Also, astronauts suffer failing digestion and intestinal functioning from the space-food diet.

The Russians will need to approve of the kimchi as an official astronaut food. In the United States, such approvals are not automatic. The National Aeronautics and Space Administration (NASA) analyze all space foods for their nutritional values, conduct sensory tests, and evaluate their performance in a zero-gravity environment.

If the processed kimchi undergoes such analyses by the Russians, it will be interesting to know the effects of the harsh processings on the nutritional values of this food.

Currently, there are hundreds of variations of kimchi. The basic form is spicy-hot, extremely pungent, fermented napa cabbage in an aromatic base. The mixture is allowed to ferment for several days and emerges as a food in which the lactic acid has created a flavorful crunchy food that is said to whet the appetite and flood the palate with agreeable tastes. The Koreans take pride in noting that kimchi fulfills all five of the basic tastes: sweet, salty, hot, sour, and bitter.

As many as five or six different kimchis serve as side dishes to a traditional meal in which the main dish consists of bland sticky rice or other grains. During the year, composition of the kimchi changes as seasonal ingredients become available. Components of kimchi differ from one region to another: shrimp are favored as an addition in Seoul; anchovies, in the south; and various fish, in the north. Spices and other flavorings vary, too. Some of the more unusual additions feature the leaves of perilla (Asian mint), mustard, or chrysanthemum; vegetables such as eggplant, wild leek (ramp), scallions, or Chinese chives; or oysters, seaweed, or pears.

Second in popularlity to napa cabbage, kimchi is fermented daikon radish kimchi, with garlic and chili pepper. This dish is reported to be sweeter and crunchier than cabbage kimchi.

Kimchi is regarded as a health-promoting dish. The Koreans believe that it regulates body fluids and intestinal fermentation, prevents constipation, and stimulates the appetite.

OTHER LACTO-FERMENTED VEGETABLES

In addition to sauerkraut, pickles, and kimchi, the lacto-fermentation process can be used with other vegetables. If you wish to prepare them at home, *Nourishing Traditions* by Sally Fallon and Mary G. Enig, mentioned earlier, is a helpful guide. If you prefer to purchase them, Bio-Lacto/Deep Root Organic Raw Cultured Vegetables, also mentioned earlier, sells lacto-fermented carrots, beets, and daikon radishes.

CHAPTER 15

Beans: Fermentation Is a Necessity

Beans are legumes, a group of plants that include, along with beans, grams, and pulses. Legumes contain protein but are either limited or lacking in certain amino acids to make them complete proteins. They also contribute carbohydrates and dietary fiber. All legumes share a common feature. Fermentation is necessary to make them fit for consumption. Raw beans contain numerous antinutrients and toxins. Cooking is not helpful, but fermentation is by reducing these substances.

FERMENTED SOYBEANS

Because the soybean is so widely used, and components of it are present in so many processed foods in the typical American diet, this bean merits more attention than other beans that are eaten less frequently, or in lesser amounts.

What are the antinutrients and toxins in soybeans? The soybean contains the following:

- **Protease inhibitors.** These substances interfere with the digestive enzyme, protease, and most notably, with trypsin. Inhibition of trypsin can lead to gastric distress, poor protein digestion, and pancreatic distress.

- **Oxalates.** These substances prevent proper calcium absorption. Oxalates are associated with kidney stones and vulvodynia (pain in the vulva).

- **Lectins.** Sometimes they are called hemagglutinins or phytoagglutinins. These substances cause red blood cells to clump together, and cause immune system reactions.

- **Phytates.** These substances impair absorption of minerals such as zinc, calcium, and iron. (Phytin from phytates is present in cereal grains, and will be discussed shortly in the next chapter.)

- **Oligosaccharides.** These sugars are responsible for bloating and gas caused by the consumption of unfermented beans. Humans lack the enzymes needed to digest these sugars.

- **Goitrogens.** Any extended use of large amounts of soybean inevitably leads to thyroid problems.

- **Saponins.** These substances bind with bile, and damage the intestinal lining.

- **Isoflavones, especially genistein and daidzein.** These two plant-derived estrogens are touted by soybean promoters as beneficial phyto-estrogens. However, as hormones, these substances are double-edged swords. They play a role in promoting, as well as retarding, the carcinogenic process.

These various antinutrients and toxins in soybeans are not eliminated by soaking or cooking. They are reduced by traditional methods of fermentation. Through the experiences of countless generations, Asian people learned to ferment soybeans and produce an astonishing number of products. Currently, in the United States, the only truly fermented soy product commonly available as a main dish is tempeh.

Tempeh

Tempeh originated in Indonesia. Traditionally, it has been home prepared daily by most families. Tempeh is fungally fermented with *Rhizopus oligosporus*. In traditional processing, dry soybeans are soaked overnight, and inoculated with a starter from an older batch, and allowed to ferment at room temperature for one or two days. The batch is consumed fresh, or preserved for future use by drying it.

K. H. Steinkraus and colleagues found that the amino acids in tempeh fermented for up to thirty hours did not differ significantly from cooked soybeans. After seventy-two hours of fermentation, most of the amino acids declined slightly. However, tryptophan (an amino acid) increased significantly up to twenty-four hours of fermentation and then declined.

After thirty-four hours of fermentation, other amino acids declined: methionine, 4 percent; and lysine, 10 percent. After sixty hours of fermentation, methionine declined 11 percent; and lysine, 24 percent. Fractions of the vitamin B complex also changed. Vitamin B_1 (thiamine) declined by 50 percent or more, but vitamin B_2 (riboflavin) more than doubled, and both vitamin B_3 (niacin) and vitamin B_{12} (cyanocobalamin) increased many fold during tempeh manufacture.

Commonly, commercial tempeh is formed into a rectangular flat loaf and can be found in the refrigerated section of health food stores.

Miso

Miso is a commonly used paste in Asian countries, and is somewhat familiar in the West. Miso's composition varies widely, depending on the ratio of its components of soybean, rice, barley, and salt. The preparation of the soybeans is similar to that used in making tempeh. The fermentation period varies from less than a month to more than a year, depending on the salt level, temperature, and ratio of soybeans to grains.

Miso is not considered to be a good vitamin source, except for riboflavin, which can be produced by a strain of *Aspergillus oryzae*.

Tamari is the liquid that accumulates when miso is ripened. Sometimes the thick miso-mash is thinned by adding more brine, as well as some wheat-containing mash. After fermentation and filtration, the resulting liquid is shoyu, a common soy sauce.

Shoyu

Known as shoyu in Japan, and *chiang-yu* in China, this is the most important fermented food product in both countries. In Japan, shoyu is made from a mixture of soybeans and wheat, in a ratio of 45:55. In China, the sauce may consist solely of soybeans, or a mixture of soybeans and a grain, with a ratio favoring the soybeans.

In the processing, the soybeans are soaked, heated with steam pressure for an hour, cooled, and mixed with roasted or steamed wheat or wheat bran. The mixture is put into a salt brine and allowed to ferment in large vats from three months to a year. The liquid is strained from the "cake" (the solids) and pasteurized. The fermentation makes the proteins, fats, and starch almost totally soluble. Occasionally, shoyu is produced as a clear product by brewing, rather than by fermenting.

Soy Sauce

Soy sauce has a long history of use as a condiment and seasoning. It is thought to have been created about 3,000 years ago in China as a byproduct of food fermentation. To preserve the food supply for winter storage, the Chinese packed meat and fish in salt, and extracted the liquid. They found that the liquid was highly flavorful and could be used as a savory seasoning. Gradually, as Buddhism became widely practiced, its vegetarian doctrine led to the substitution of soybeans and grains instead of meat and fish to produce soy sauce.

Soy sauce was introduced into Japan during the Heian period (794 to 1185) by a Zen priest who had studied in China. Subsequently, soy sauce production thrived in Japan.

Early soy sauce was based on miso, and often was thick and sweet. This was a forerunner of present-day tamari products. Soy sauce became an indispensable component of Japanese cuisine. Sauces always contain soy, but grain additions may include wheat, barley, or rice.

There is a great deal of difference in the quality of soy sauces. There is standard soy sauce, a type intended for export from Japan, and then there is imperial soy sauce, restricted to limited domestic consumption.

Currently, Kikkoman is the largest manufacturer of soy sauce in the world. The main fermentation plant is in Noda, Japan, and there are additional plants in Japan, as well as in the United States, the Netherlands, Singapore, Taiwan, and China. Kikkoman produces soy sauces solely from soybeans and wheat. For the standard soy sauce, the soybeans are from the United States and the wheat is from Canada. For the imperial soy sauce, both the soybeans and the wheat are derived exclusively from Japanese-grown crops.

The process for making the soy sauces begins with the soybeans being steamed to softness, drained of excessive moisture, and mashed with roasted and finely ground wheat. The mixture is inoculated with *A. oryzae* and then spread onto wooden trays. Later, the mixture is transferred to a culture room and put into giant cedarwood vats. Each vat holds enough liquid to fill 5,000 bottles. The vats are painted orange-red, the traditional color of Shinto, a major religion in Japan. The moisture content of the mixture and its temperature are monitored constantly. When the mixture has become dry it is inoculated with a saline solution of koji mash. (Koji is a fungus used in wine fermenation.) The mixture remains in the vats, bubbling and fermenting for a year. Yeasts are added to assist in the maturation process.

After the full year of fermentation, small batches of the mash are transferred into nylon sleeves. They are forced through wood presses where the liquid is drained, then heated, and pasteurized to stabilize the color and aroma before being bottled. Although the standard and the imperial soy sauces may have similar appearances, the imperial soy sauce is reported to have a far greater intensity of flavor. Currently, with the royal family's permission, the imperial soy sauce is sold in a few selected Japanese shops.

Fermented Foods and Vitamin K_2

Vitamin K has long been known as the blood-clotting vitamin. Until recently, it was thought to be a single vitamin. Then, it was discovered that the vitamin has different fractions, and each has different functions.

Humans and other animals obtain vitamin K_1 (phylloquinone) from the green tissues of plants. However, we now know that a portion of vitamin K_1 is converted into vitamin K_2 (menaquinone-7).

Vitamin K_1 is used, preferentially, by the liver to activate blood-clotting proteins. Vitamin K_2 activates protein-dependent vitamins A and D by conferring upon them the physical ability to bind calcium. Vitamin K_2 is used, preferentially, by tissues to place calcium, appropriately, in bones and teeth and to prevent calcium from being placed, inappropriately, in soft tissues.

In addition to food sources from leafy greens, vitamin K_2 also is produced by beneficial flora in the gastrointestinal tract, as well as by lactic acid bacteria that produce fermented foods. Thus, fermented foods contain vitamin K_2.

As recently as 2006, the first listing of the vitamin K_2-containing foods was compiled in the United States. A team of researchers from the U.S. Department of Agriculture (USDA) and Tufts University, led by S. J. Elder, found that the best sources of vitamin K_2 are from animal-derived foods and from fermented foods.

The fats of grass-fed animals are especially good sources of vitamin K_2. For vegetarians who would shun animal fats, natto, the Japanese fermented food, is a good source of vitamin K_2.

Although traditional soy sauce has been produced by fermentation, a more recent technique that is cheaper, quicker, but harsh is to produce the soy sauce by acid hydrolysis. Soy sauce made in Vietnam by acid hydrolysis was seized in 2002 when it was imported by Australia. The Australian-New Zealand Food Authority found that the product contained cancer-causing chloropropanols at extremely high levels. The lesson to be drawn from this episode is to read soy sauce labels carefully to make certain that the products are produced through fermentation. Avoid inexpensive soy sauce, which likely is produced by acid hydrolysis.

Natto

Natto is another soybean-based fermented food widely used in Japan. The process of making natto is similar to that with tempeh, except that natto is inoculated with a bacterium rather than with a mold. The fermentation is done with *Bacillus subtilis.* The fermentation process produces two vitamin B fractions: thiamine and riboflavin.

An analysis of natto by T. Sano found that the thiamine and riboflavin increased threefold over that of the original soybeans, and vitamin B_{12} increased nearly fivefold.

Tofu

Tofu is a readily recognized soy product to most Americans, and is available nationwide in supermarkets. Although the common perception is that tofu is a fermented food, it is not. Rather, it is a coagulated food.

To prepare tofu, soybeans are ground or milled with water to form soybean "milk." It is strained to remove the insoluble solids. A curd is formed by coagulating the heated liquid with a solution of a salt of calcium or magnesium. The curd is formed in a cheese mold lined with cheesecloth. The liquid is drained away. The resulting tofu is a bland fiber-free product consisting of about 80 percent water, 10 percent protein, and 4 percent fats. The curd contains only about 40 percent of the protein in the original soybeans, and retains only about 20 percent of the original thiamine, riboflavin, and niacin, according to the findings by C. D. Miller and colleagues.

If the salt of calcium is chosen rather than the salt of magnesium, the calcium content of tofu is about 170 milligrams per 100 grams of tofu, an amount that is somewhat higher than in cow's milk. However, there is no assurance that the calcium is absorbed and utilized as well.

Home-Prepared Tofu May Not Be Safe

The Centers for Disease Control and Prevention (CDC) noted that home-made tofu and other bean products that are fermented are the most common foods causing botulism in China. From 1958 to 1989, home-fermented bean products were responsible for 63 percent of some 2,000 botulism cases in China.

In December 2006, the first incidence of botulism caused by eating home-prepared tofu was reported in the United States. The Orange County Health Care Agency and the California Department of Health Services were notified of two potential cases of foodborne botulism in an elderly Asian couple who had prepared tofu at home. Laboratory analysis of the tofu identified both *Clostridium botulinum type A* and its toxin in the tofu samples, which had a pH of 6.8. Botulinum spores can germinate and grow in a pH less than 4.6.

Sufu

Sufu, a product of tofu, but unlike tofu, is a mold-fermented product. It is inoculated with *Actinomucor elegans*, and fermented from three to seven days. Then, it is aged and stored in brine to which may be added flavoring substances such as wine, fermented rice mash, or hot peppers. During the aging process, the proteins and fats of the soybean curd are digested by the enzymes of the mold's mycelia (threadlike strands produced by fungi).

OTHER FERMENTED LEGUMES

The use of fermented legumes is popular throughout Indonesia. Two of the most common products are idli and ontjom.

Idli

Black gram, a leguminous plant such as chickpeas (garbanzos) or mung beans, is consumed commonly in Asia, especially in southern India. The black gram is soaked in water for six hours, drained, and ground to a paste, along with parboiled or soaked rice. The proportions used to make idli, a popular savory cake, may be equal amounts of gram and rice, but may vary. The mixture is inoculated with *Leuconostoc mesenteroides*, and allowed to ferment for fifteen hours or longer. Analyses vary, but

R. Rajalakshmi and K. Vanaja reported that both thiamine and riboflavin had a twofold to threefold increase in fermented black gram over the original unfermented black gram. The amino acid methionine was 20 percent greater.

Ontjom

Ontjom are red or white press cakes made from peanuts, a legume. Sometimes carbohydrates such as tapioca or potato are added. The press cakes are fermented by *Rhizopus* or *Neurospora sitophila*. They are consumed commonly in southern India. Oncom is a similar peanut press cake consumed in Indonesia. It, too, is fermented by the fungus *N. sitophila*.

THE OVERUSE OF SOY

Because soy is so overused in American food products, it has become one of the eight major allergens in the diet. Even milk-allergic infants, placed on soy-based formulations, become allergic to soy.

In the West, we should have learned the necessity of fermenting the soybean to make it suitable for consumption. During World War II, many of the fermentation plants in Asia were destroyed by bombings. There were great food shortages. As a humanitarian gesture, the United States shipped soybeans to Asian countries. Despite the lean times, the Asians were reluctant to consume the soybeans in an unfermented form. Gradually, American officials came to understand that the Asians considered fermentation of soybeans a necessity. We helped rebuild the destroyed fermentation plants, and Asians accepted the subsequent soybean shipments with appreciation.

THE UPSIDE OF FERMENTED SOYBEANS

Researchers at the National University of Singapore found that dark soy sauce derived from fermented soybeans, which is used widely in East Asia, may prove to be a potent agent in combating human cell damage by free radicals. The research team, led by Professor Barry Halliwell, found that fermented soybean sauce was about ten times more effective as an antioxidant than red wine, and about 150 times more effective than vitamin C. Also, the study showed that the soy sauce improved blood flow up to 50 percent in the hours after consumption of the sauce. Regarding the sauce, Halliwell was quoted in *Food Processing's Wellness Foods* (Aug 2006) as saying, "There's a preventive aspect, showing that it may potentially slow down the rate of cardiovascular and neuro-degenerative diseases."

Fermented soybean products are being offered to food processors as their value becomes better recognized. One product is a flavor enhancer, Soyarome, manufactured by Gist-brocade in King of Prussia, Pennsylvania. This product is made by proprietary fermentation and enzyme technologies. The product is intended to flavor vegetables, dairy foods, and spices. If used in products, it can be labeled as "fermented soy flour."

Fermented soybeans are the raw materials in dietary supplements. One commercial product is offered as a nutritional adjuvant for cancer patients. Haelan 951 Fermented Soy, a beverage produced by Haelan Products in Woodinville, Washington, is described as a nitrogenation process that hydrolyzes many of the soybean proteins into bioactive amino acids and compounds consisting of various fermentation metabolites of substances present in soybeans. The process is reported to break down these substances to smaller molecules that are more bioavailable. (For more information, see www.haelan951.com.)

Another fermented soy dietary aid, in tablet form, is Sano-Gastril, produced by Allergy Research Group in San Leandro, California. This probiotic is fermented with a strain of *Lactobacillus bulgaricus 51* rather than by fungal fermentation. The product is reported to contain bioactive compounds that are beneficial for gastrointestinal health.

BEANS AND THE GI TRACT

All beans are notorious producers of gastrointestinal bloating and gas. A group of food scientists, including Marisela Granito at Simón Bolivar University in Caracas, Venezuela, and colleagues in France and Spain, discovered that fermentation eliminated the compounds that cause humans to produce bloating and gas. By fermenting beans up to ninety-six hours, the researchers were able to remove up to 95 percent of the offending compounds. The researchers noted that the fermentation process offered an additional bonus, by increasing protein digestibility and carbohydrate availability (*Journal of Science of Food and Agriculture*, 2003).

Some types of beans are more gas producing than others because of the naturally occurring oligosaccharides contained in the beans. These are sugars that require an enzyme to digest them. This enzyme is found normally in the human gut, but some people have insufficient amounts of the enzyme.

Beans with high amounts of oligosaccharides include Great Northern, pinto, black, red kidney, soy, and navy. Beans with lesser amounts of these sugars include the black-eye pea, lima bean, chickpea , and lentil.

The USDA suggests boiling unsoaked beans for two minutes, followed by soaking them for an hour, discarding the water, and cooking them in a fresh supply of water.

Soaking beans leaches out some of the oligosaccharides. There are some additional procedures that people have found to be helpful. Soak the beans overnight, and then discard the water. Add fresh water several times, and discard it each time. Some people claim that helpful measures are longer soakings and slower cooking of the beans.

Some people add sunflower oil, dill weed, rosemary, parsley, or the cilantro-like epazote (found in Latino markets and in some specialty stores) to the soaking water. They claim that these additions reduce the gaseous qualities in the beans.

A commercial product, Beano, widely available, is intended to reduce the bloating and gas after bean consumption. The product contains an enzyme needed to digest the oligosaccharides. However, the best solution to reduce bloating and gas from beans is to use them in a fermented form.

CHAPTER 16

Cereal Grains: Improved Through Fermentation

The search for antimicrobial substances that are effective against food spoilage and pathogenic organisms has increased greatly due to a growing interest to enhance food safety by use of biopreservatives. There is interest, especially, in finding substances that are active against Gram-negative bacteria, yeasts, and molds, many of which cause disease. Certain microorganisms, used for centuries in fermented foods, can serve as a safe source of hitherto unconsidered antimicrobial aids. Many of these substances are present in fermented cereal grains.

FERMENTED CEREAL GRAINS

As noted earlier in the book, fermented cereal grains have been used extensively in traditional diets: millet, corn, and teff in different regions of Africa; rice, in Asia; and corn and rice, in Latin America. Fermentation was achieved simply by exposing moistened crushed or ground grain to wild yeasts present in the air.

In modern times, studies reveal the wisdom of eating wholegrains only after they have undergone fermentation. A component in the fiber of cereal grains, called phytin, binds dietary minerals such as zinc and calcium. Zinc binding is more of a problem than calcium binding, because calcium is provided in other foods. Zinc is more difficult to supply, especially because it is stripped from foods in the refining process. Such foods prevail, but many Americans do not eat zinc-rich foods. To some degree, many Americans are zinc deficient.

Fermenting porridge or leavening bread degrades the phytin, and allows the nutrients to be utilized. Fermentation also improves the grain's digestibility. (See "Fermenting Porridge at Home" on page 146 and "Making a Sourdough Starter" on page 148.)

If cereal grains form a large portion of the diet, unfermented porridge or unleavened bread can lead to health problems. For example, severe zinc deficiency can lead to mental retardation in children.

A dramatic episode in the Middle East demonstrated this truth. Poor children ate large quantities of unleavened wheat bread. They showed signs of severe zinc deficiency. The condition was stopped simply by switching the children to leavened bread.

Fermented Corn

Pozol is an indigenous fermented corn dough used in Mexico since the time of a flourishing Mayan civilization. The fermented pozol displays a broad spectrum of antimicrobial activity, identified by C. G. Sanchez-Fernandez and L. L. McKay, from the Department of Food Science and Nutrition at the University of Minnesota in St. Paul. The researchers isolated *Agrobacterium azotophilum* from pozol. The bacterium displayed a spectrum of inhibitory activity against pathogens. The researchers then isolated another strain, *A. azotophilum* CS93, also from pozol, which was even more effective. Both strains were able to inhibit many important microorganisms, such as *Aspergillus* spp. (several species) and *Fusarium* sp. (one specie); yeasts such as *Saccharomycin* sp. and *Kluyveromyces* sp.; Gram-positive bacteria such as *Bacillus cereus, Staphylococcus aureus,* and *Listeria monocytogenes;* and gram-negative bacteria such as *Escherichia coli, Salmonella* sp. and *Pseudomonas* spp. The antimicrobial substances could be valuable as natural biopreservatives against both gram-negative and gram-positive bacteria, as well as against spoilage molds and yeasts.

Fermented Rice

Sierra rice is a dietary staple in Ecuador. It is made by fermenting rice with a mold, *Aspergillus flavus.* In laboratory analysis, the vitamin B_2 (riboflavin) in the fermented rice increased twofold over that in the untreated rice. When rice was fermented with *Bacillus subtilis,* the vitamin B_2 increased fivefold over that of the untreated rice. This example shows the wisdom of the traditional practice of fermenting cereal grains. They are not only rendered more digestible, but also sometimes increase their nutritional offerings.

Fermented Barley

Barley has gained a reputation as a healthy wholegrain that contributes to the American diet. Currently, fermented barley extract is offered to food processors by Barley Fermentation Technologies in St. Louis, Missouri, with headquarters in Fukuoka, Japan.

The barley extract is made from a byproduct of alcoholic distillation of Japanese *shōchū*. The extract consists of peptides, amino acids including gamma aminobutyric acid (GABA), oligosaccharides, and citric acid. To create the fermented barley extract, shochu lees (the dregs) serve as the raw materials. They are broken down by enzymes in koji during the shochu distillation and fermentation of shochu yeast. The shochu lees are purified and then concentrated into an extract.

According to Barley Fermentation Technologies, the shochu lees have been shown to improve lipid metabolism. They might have a protective effect on the liver. In animal studies, the shochu lees showed beneficial antioxidant activity.

The fermented barley extract is offered to food processors, with suggested uses in breads, snack foods, pizza dough, pastas, energy drinks, sauces, and condiments. The extract is reported to "round out and heighten the flavor" of food products.

Fermented Wheat Protein

A fermented wheat protein product is available to food processors from Kikkoman as a flavor enhancer replacement for the controversial compounds of monosodium glutamate (MSG) and hydrolyzed vegetable protein (HVP). The product can be listed on the ingredient panel of food products as "fermented wheat protein." Kikkoman reported that the fermented wheat protein product would be useful with meats, poultry, seafoods, dressings, dry mixes, and seasoning blends.

Fermented Wheat Germ

A concentrated extract from fermented wheat germ has been shown to have immune modulating effects and potential anticancer effects, too. These findings were drawn from in vitro studies of cells, animal experiments, and clinical trials with humans. All of the studies were reported in peer-reviewed journals.

The concentrated extract, Avemar, is a patented process, resulting from the initial interest in wheat germ for medical therapy by the Nobel scientist, Albert Szent-Györgyi. He studied various extracts of the wheat plant for their immune-enhancing effects. His studies were continued by a fellow Hungarian biologist, Dr. Máté Hidvégi, who developed a technique of fermenting wheat germ. He found that the extract has multiple mechanisms of activity. This feature may make it possible for the extract to benefit a range of health disorders. The extract, now patented, has a record of safety, and has been designated as GRAS (Generally Recognized as Safe). The extract, already in use throughout Europe, in parts of the Middle East, and Africa, now is available in the United States as a dietary supplement named Avé from American BioSciences.

Avemar has been shown to be effective against all cancer cell lines tested, including breast, prostate, lung, pancreatic, lymphomic, and leukemic. Animal studies showed the extract to be a cancer preventative, and to have antimetastatic properties. In human clinical trials, the extract showed highly significant therapeutic effects against primary colorectal cancer, stage III melanoma, and stages III and IV oral cancers. Also, the extract improved the quality of life for cancer patients. The extract was able to reduce side effects, such as suppression of immune function, resulting from conventional cytotoxic cancer therapies.

SOURDOUGH FOR LEAVENING

Unleavened bread was probably a common feature of the late Stone Age, made from wild grains with their characteristically adherent husks that

Fermenting Porridge at Home

Take advantage of traditional wisdom and ferment your porridge. Although many traditional porridges were fermented for days to achieve strong tartness, the process can be shortened, with no perceptible tartness in the porridge, yet achieve the goals of reduced phytin and increased digestibility. If you plan to eat porridge for breakfast, begin preparation the night before.

Soak a wholegrain such as brown rice, wild rice, millet, quinoa, amaranth, teff, barley, undegerminated corn grits, steel-cut oatmeal or bulgur overnight in water (about one part grain to two parts water) with one or two teaspoonsful of liquid whey from yogurt. Or, add a teaspoonful of plain powdered whey sold in health food stores. Allow the mixture to soak in the pot at room temperature. In the morning, cook the porridge in the soaking liquid. Cooking time varies, from about ten to twenty minutes, depending on the type of grain.

were difficult to detach, unless the grain was parched. Surviving versions of unleavened bread include the flat bread, tortilla, Indian johnnycake, chapati, Chinese pancake, matzo, and some crackers.

There is evidence that leavened bread developed in Egypt around 4,000 BC. It evolved after Egyptians selected a cultivated wheat variety that could be husked readily. The process of leavening soon followed, probably with bread dough left too long in a warm place, and fermented with wild yeasts in the air. The Egyptians found the leavened bread agreeable tasting. Perhaps, too, they noted that it was more digestible than the unleavened bread.

At some point in time, it was discovered that if a portion of the leavened dough was taken out of the mix, it could be kept to ferment the subsequent batch. Such leavening is known as sourdough.

Sourdough-leavened bread appeals to consumers because of its agreeable flavor and aroma. In times and places where other leavening agents were unavailable, sourdough was prized. The men who sought to make their fortunes in the Klondike Goldrush (1897–1898) not only packed axes and pans among their gear, but also included a supply of sourdough starter. It was reported that the men guarded their precious supply of sourdough by sleeping with it to provide enough body warmth to keep it from freezing. Sourdough was bartered and sometimes stolen. Sourdough became so closely associated with the men that they became known as "Sourdoughs."

In more recent times, sourdough is still valued. The most prestigious Parisian bakers produce sourdough-leavened products. San Francisco is famous for its sourdough breads. Yet, the San Francisco-like sourdough breads produced elsewhere only approximate the real San Francisco product. Among several factors, it may be a question of wild yeasts in the atmosphere that differ from one location to another. This feature played a role in an episode in cheesemaking. A company moved its plant from one location to another. The technologists were puzzled. The ingredients were the same, the process was the same, and the equipment was the same. But the cheese was different. The technologists had to scrape some of the yeasts present in the old plant and inoculate them in the new plant to reclaim the characteristics of the formerly produced cheese. Likewise with sourdough.

Sourdough varies from batch to batch, depending on the wild yeasts in the air, as well as the ratio of ingredients, temperature, time, and other factors. Even the yeast that settle on walls within a bakery may be crucial. Annemarie Colbin, founder of the Natural Gourmet Cookery School and Institute for Food and Health in New York City, relates a true story about sourdough bread. A bakery was renowned for its sourdough bread. Then, as a sanitary measure, the health department required the bakery to paint the interior walls. The bread lost its distinctive flavor after the paint cov-

Making a Sourdough Starter

It is easy to make homemade sourdough. There are two basic methods.

- **Method 1.** Reserve a cup of dough or batter before the remainder is baked or cooked. It is preferable to use dough or batter before salt is added to it. Place the dough or batter in a clean glass jar or crock. Cap or cover it and allow it to remain at room temperature for several days. Depending on the temperature, the sourdough will smell pleasantly sour and will be ready to be added to dough or batter. If the sourdough is ready to be used before you are ready to use it, refrigerate it. The lower temperature will slow down the souring process.

    If you do not plan to use the sourdough within a few days, freeze or dry it, and reactivate it at a later date. To freeze the sourdough, place it in an airtight container and store it in the freezer, until you wish to use it. To revive, simply thaw it. To dry the sourdough, add enough flour to shape it into a ball, and place it in a bag of flour. In the dried form, the yeast goes into a spore stage and remains inert for a long time. Revive the yeast to an active stage by adding water and placing it in a warm location.

- **Method 2.** In a clean glass jar, soak one-half teaspoon of dried yeast granules in one-half cup of warm (not hot) water until it froths. Add a cup of wholegrain flour and one-half cup of additional warm water. Stir, and cap the jar. Store it at room temperature. Allow the mixture to rise and fall for two to three days until it attains the desired tartness. Then, add the sourdough to dough or batter, and remember to reserve some starter for the next batch. Refrigerate the starter in a glass jar.

With care, sourdough starter should continue indefinitely. However, if it develops any unusual appearance or odor, discard it, and start anew.

ered the yeast. Reluctantly, the bakery discontinued making its famous sourdough bread.

GRAIN-BASED FERMENTED TONICS

Some traditional fermented beverages are based on cereal grains rather than milk. They have a low-alcoholic content, and have been regarded as tonics.

Kvass

Kvass (also *kvas*) has been made in Russia from stale bread or from a cereal grain such as barley, oats, rye, or wheat. Kvass is made by incomplete fermentation of alcohol and lactic acid over a brief period of several days. Kvass has been an important staple in the Russian diet as a daily drink. Traditionally, it has been made in the home. Also, it has been sold by street vendors in towns and at markets.

Kvass has been most popular in central Russia and Siberia. There are many regional variations. In Ukraine, kvass has been made from fermented beets, and has been used not only as a low-alcoholic beverage, but also as a stock for soups and stews. In some areas, kvass has been flavored with berries or fruits.

Rejuvelac

Rejuvelac (a word coined by the late raw-food enthusiast Ann Wigmore) is another fermented tonic based on cereal grain. Wigmore claimed that the drink was a digestive aid, with its enzymes, beneficial bacteria, and vitamins. It is made by soaking any whole grain in cool water, in a ratio of one-part grain to three-parts water. After storage at room temperature for twenty-four hours, the liquid is poured into a clean glass jar, covered with cheesecloth, and stored at room temperature for about two days to allow the liquid to ferment. Then, it is ready to drink. Any unused portion can be refrigerated for future use. Meanwhile, the soaked grains can be cooked as a cereal. More water needs to be added.

Kombucha

Kombucha is another fermented tonic, but it is not based on milk, grain, or other foods. Kombucha's origin is reported to be from Russia in the distant past. It was used in other eastern European countries as well as in the Far East, in Japan, China, and Indonesia. In China, it was mentioned as early as 221 BC during the Tsin Dynasty. Kombucha is known by different names, including Manchurian tea, tea kvass, tea fungus, chainyi grib, teeschwamm, teewass, wunderpilz, hongo, cajnij, and fungus japonicus.

It is made by culturing a water solution of sugar and black tea. Both substances are converted by a culturing fungus, acetic-acid producing *Acetobacter* sp., accompanied by two yeasts. The fungus and yeasts form a symbiotic combination to make the culture, which sometimes is called a "mushroom." The resulting fermented drink, kombucha, is somewhat reminiscent of apple cider in taste.

Kombucha is reported to be a salutary tonic, and a natural detoxifier. Glucuronic acid, its main beneficial component, is a natural acid that binds to environmental and metabolic toxins and excretes them via the kidneys. Also, glucuronic acid is the building block of a group of important polysaccharides that include hyaluronic acid (a basic component of connective tissue), chondroitin sulfate (a basic component of cartilage, and currently popular as a dietary supplement to ease arthritic conditions), and mucoitin sulfuric acid (a building block of the stomach lining and of the vitreous humor of the eye).

In fermenting kombucha, the starter doubles with each batch. You may find someone who has a thriving culture and is willing to share some of it. Also, the culture is available commercially, from GEM Cultures in Lakewood, Washington (www.gemcultures.com). Kombucha boosters maintain a worldwide Kombucha Exchange at www.kombu.de. Kombucha "mothers" are available without cost other than shipping charges.

Because kombucha is fermented, in part, with yeasts, this tonic may not be suitable for individuals who have yeast infections.

Conclusion

Fermentation has benefited humans in the past by providing a safe means of storing foods and beverages, increasing their nutrients, and improving their flavors. Fermention has also benefited humans by providing a means of maintaining and restoring health.

Unfortunately, the tradition of fermentation, appreciated by our ancestors, had all but disappeared in the industrialized world. The growing interest in probiotics makes fermentation more important than ever. Fermentation allows us to preserve foods safely without resorting to toxic substances (such as chemical preservatives) or to processings of dubious safety (such as the radiation-preservation of foods). Therapeutically, fermented foods such as yogurt act gently and effectively to alleviate health disorders such as chronic yeast infections or chronic constipation. The value of fermented foods to combat infectious agents is constant, whereas microbes learn to resist antibiotic drugs, and the drugs themselves become less and less effective. Also, eating fermented foods strengthens the immune system. Fermented foods become instruments of preventive medicine.

APPENDIX A

Probiotics as Dietary Supplements

As dietary supplements have proliferated, it was inevitable that probiotics would be swept along with the trend. These products have become so numerous that, unfortunately, the word probiotic to many people is synonymous with supplements rather than with traditional sources of cultured foods. As with other dietary supplements, the probiotics should not replace foods, but rather be regarded as possible useful adjuncts.

Probiotic supplements are intended mainly for intestinal health. Judging by the number of over-the-counter products sold for heartburn, gas, diarrhea, laxation, and other intestinal ailments, gastrointestinal (GI) health is no small matter for Americans.

Probiotic supplements are available as tablets, capsules, powders, and in liquid form. Casein- and gluten-free products are available. All probiotic supplements are not alike, nor do they have similar therapeutic values. The supplements need to contain the correct strains, in the correct amounts, and in the correct formulation under correct conditions for the intended use. This is a tall order.

SELECTING THE CORRECT STRAIN

Lactic acid bacteria have had a long history of safe use in cultured dairy foods. However, some probiotic dietary supplements contain certain bacteria that have no history of safe use in humans or in other animals. According to S. K. Dash of UAS Laboratories in Minnetonka, Minnesota, some probiotic supplements contain soil bacteria that are not normal inhabitants of the human GI tract, and are potentially pathogenic. Dash recommends that bacteria species used in probiotic supplements be limited to those on the FDA's GRAS list, such as *L. acidophilus* and some strains of *Bifidobacteria*. According to Dash, any new bacterial culture with

153

no history of prior safe use in humans should be subjected to toxicological studies prior to its use in probiotic supplements. Also, he believes that the bacterial strains used in quality supplements should play important roles in

- colonizing within the intestinal, respiratory, and urogenital tracts

- benefiting cholesterol metabolism

- inhibiting carcinogenesis, both directly and indirectly, by stimulating the immune system

- metabolizing lactose, calcium absorption, and vitamin synthesis

- reducing yeast and vaginal infection

- alleviating constipation and diarrheal diseases

- relieving gastritis and ulcerations

- helping to reduce acne and other skin problems

Additionally, Dash recommends that the probiotic supplement should adhere to the intestinal walls, and be able to proliferate. The probiotic strain must be proven to survive stomach acidity in humans. It should be able to produce natural antibiotics, lactic acid, and hydrogen peroxide in order to inhibit pathogenic bacteria.

Not all strains of *L. acidophilus* and other probiotics are acid-resistant. For the probiotic to be effective, acid-resistant strains of bacteria must be chosen. Enteric coating of bacteria is a poor and unproven substitute for actual acid resistance, reports Dash. No studies have been conducted to prove their usefulness. On the contrary, Dash suggests that by coating live cultures with a protective layer, the culture's viability may be *reduced or even be killed*.

Well-studied strains of *Lactobacillus* and *Bifidobacteria* survive stomach acidity and reach the intestine where they can be beneficial. Frequently, hardy strains of these bacteria are used in probiotic supplements.

The amount of colony forming units (CFUs) or live organisms at the time of manufacture depends on the type of bacteria. The CFUs should be in the billions. Heat, moisture, oxygen, time, and possibly enteric coating, may all decrease survival of the bacteria.

In some cases, probiotic supplements may deliver less than they promise. According to ConsumerLab.com in White Plains, New York, an independent laboratory that analyzes products, nearly one-third of the probiotics they sampled contained less than 1 percent of the claimed numbers of live bacteria.

Another study, led by Todd Klaenhammer, director of Southeast Dairy Food Research Center at North Carolina State University, Raleigh, examined twenty probiotic products sold to consumers. All products were claimed to contain *L. acidophilus*. The team sequenced the 16S DNA genes of the products to make a true identification. Only eight of the twenty products examined contained the organism claimed on the label. The rest included organisms such as *L. gallinarum, L. delbrueckii,* or *Pediococcus pentosacceus.* The researchers fingerprinted the eight *L. acidophilus*-containing products and found that they all had very similar genetic content.

ADDITIONAL CONSIDERATIONS WITH PROBIOTIC SUPPLEMENTS

As with yogurt, are single or mixed strains preferable in probiotic supplements? Some probiotic supplements with mixed strains may be unsafe, warns Dash. Many of the strains being used have no safe history in human health and nutrition. Some bacteria may be antagonistic to each other, and may alter the gut flora in an undesirable way. More may not be better. On the contrary, a few selected cultures have been proven beneficial; almost all of the others have yet to be proven.

Dash's warnings were prescient. By 2008, experimental therapy with a mixture of probiotics revealed potential hazards. In a clinical trial at Utrecht University in the Netherlands, 296 patients with acute pancreatitis were given a mixture of six presumably benign bacteria by feeding tube in an attempt to prevent infection. One of the lead researchers, Hein Gooszen, announced the unanticipated results: the death of twenty-four patients from multiple organ failures. There was speculation that the mixture of bacterial strains might have triggered an unforeseen immune reaction. In most previous trials, only one or two bacterial strains of probiotics had been used in test-tube and animal experiments, and they had inhibited the growth of most common pathogens that cause pancreatic complications.

The manufacturing process plays a vital role in the viability of the culture in a probiotic supplement. Quality control is essential. Without it, the product will not contain the same strain, a similar number of bacteria, the same level of high viability of the bacteria, batch after batch. Nor will it produce, consistently, the same good results. Quality control also should ensure that the product has not been contaminated with harmful bacteria during the manufacturing process.

The consumer should have some indication that the supplement has been tested for its viability at the time of manufacture. The number of viable cells should be guaranteed as CFUs per gram at the time of packaging the product. Probiotic supplements should contain from 2 to 5 billion CFUs per gram for daily consumption to have any chance of offering significant beneficial effects.

Probiotic supplements should be handled like yogurts and cheeses, as products that require refrigeration in order not to spoil or lose their integrity. The probiotic supplements should be stored and shipped refrigerated at 40°F before reaching consumers.

Is there a preferred packaging for probiotic supplements? As mentioned earlier, probiotics are anaerobic organisms that live in the absence of oxygen. Exposure to air is undesirable. Glass is preferable to plastic for the container. Glass is inert; plastic is porous. During prolonged storage, probiotic supplements packaged in plastic can lose their potency.

Prebiotics are substances that selectively provide the growth of healthy intestinal bacteria such as *Lactobacillus* and *Bifidobacteria* at the expense of putrefactive bacteria such as *Clostridia*, and other coliforms. Some probiotic supplements contain added prebiotics such as fructooligosaccharides (FOS) to provide this function.

Is one form of probiotic better than others? Capsules and tablets may be a better form than powder for several reasons. It is difficult to measure an exact dosage with loose powder. Each time the container is opened, the contents are exposed to oxygen, and possibly to contaminants in the air. The powder becomes oxidized and it is exposed to humidity. The spoon used to measure the powder, if not sterilized, may contaminate the powder. For these reasons, the powder form of the probiotic supplement tends to deteriorate more rapidly than with capsules and tablets. Liquid probiotic supplements normally do not survive more than a few weeks. Another disadvantage with the liquid form is that microorganisms in a liquid medium can mutate and change.

LABEL INFORMATION SHOULD BE INFORMATIVE

The label information on probiotic supplements should identify the specie and strain of the probiotic bacterium contained in the supplement. For example, a listing might be *Lactobacillus* (specie) followed by *acidophilus* (strain). Some may identify specie, and strain followed by sub-strain, such as *L. acidophilus* GG.

The label should state the minimum number of viable cells per gram of the bacterium at the time of manufacture. Also, there should be an expiration date, directions for use, and storage information. Although some probiotic supplements may not require refrigeration, it is best to store both unopened and opened containers of these products in the refrigerator. After the container is opened, make certain to close it tightly after each opening.

Probiotics are sold to consumers as dietary supplements, and patented strains of probiotics are sold to food and beverage manufacturers for use as ingredients in so-called functional foods. A measure of the booming business is reflected in the sales figures for probiotic products in the United States. By 2002, sales of these products had reached $1.4 billion annually.

In recent years, patented probiotic strains of bacteria have been developed in many areas of the globe, including North America, Europe, Asia, and the Pacific Rim.

In the United States, Biogaia in Raleigh, North Carolina, provides two patented strains of *Lactobacillus reuteri: L. reuteri* MM2 and *L. reuteri* SD2112. Nebraska Cultures in Lincoln, Nebraska, sells *L. acidophilus* DDS. Rhodia in Madison, Wisconsin, offers *L. acidophilus* NC FM®.

In Canada, Institut Rosell produces *L. rhamnosus* R0052 and *L. acidophilus* R0011. Urex Biotech provides *L. rhamnosus* GR-1 and *L. fermentum* RC-14.

In Europe, patented probiotic strains are made in various countries. In Sweden, Arla Dairy produces *L. paracasei* F19. Essum AB offers *Lactococcus lactis* L1A and *L. rhamnosus* LB21. Probi AB provides *L. plantarum* 299V and *L. rhamnosus* 271. In Denmark, Chr. Hansen sells *L. acidophilus* LA-1 and *L. paracasei* CRL 431. In Finland, Valio Dairy provides *L. rhamnosus* GG. In France, Lacteol Laboratory produces *L. acidophilus* LB. In Switzerland, Nestlé offers two strains of *L. johnsonii: L. johnsonii* La1 and *L. johnsonii* Lj1.

In Japan, Morinaga Milk Industry Company produces *Bifidobacillus longum* BB536, and Yakult offers *B. breve* strain *Yakult* and *L. casei Shirota*.

In New Zealand, the New Zealand Dairy Board produces *B. lactis* HN019 (DR10).

Lactobacillus and *Bifidobacteria* are most commonly associated with probiotic activity. However, *Escherichia, Enterococcus,* and *Saccharomyces* strains have shown probiotic activity. In a patented form, U.S.-based Bio Balance Corporation entered *E. coli* strain BU-230-98.

According to Kantha Shelke, contributing editor of *Food Processing* both consumers and manufacturers "are becoming increasingly aware that the benefits of probiotics go beyond the gut and, as a result, the marketplace is bound to see a wide range of new probiotic products." At the same time, Shelke noted that "Commercial interests develop and guard their microbiological strains zealously."

APPENDIX B

Bioactive Probiotic Components in Milk

Milk contains a surprising number of bioactive components with probiotic activity. Among them are proteins, peptides, enzymes, and fats. Some comprise a small amount in milk's composition, but they play important roles.

PROBIOTICS IN WHEY AND WHEY PROTEINS

Whey is a byproduct of fermented milk products. Formerly, whey was considered to be a waste disposal problem for cheese producers. A hundred pounds of milk yields only about ten pounds of cheese. The remaining ninety pounds is whey. Only a small portion of the whey was utilized as food. Some was fed to hogs and used to fertilize fields. Frequently, much of the whey was dumped into rivers and created serious pollution. Then, the use of low-cost, highly nutritious dried whey came to be regarded as a useful addition to foreign aid programs. The market expanded further when it was discovered that whey could be a profitable addition to specific foods. Soon, whey's nutritional values became better recognized, and perhaps more importantly, whey's bioactive qualities became recognized as valuable. Some health food stores sell powdered whey. (Avoid the products in which whey is merely an ingredient.)

Individual whey proteins have different bioactivity. For example, beta (ß)-lactoglobulin is a retinol-binding protein that is thought to bind vitamin A and supply this vitamin to the newborn infant. Both ß-lactoglobulin and alpha (α)-lactalbumin influence mitotic activity (cell division) in the mammary gland, and have the ability to synthesize protein. The main biological role for α-lactalbumin is to synthesize lactose in the mammary gland. There is some evidence that α-lactalbumin has antitumor effects. Unfortunately, ß-lactoglobulin is the major allergen in milk.

Whey protein concentrate, derived from colostrum (the premilk present in the first four days after birth that is richly complex with important immune-protective compounds; to learn more, see Appendix C next) is associated with immunoglobulin (Ig) concentration. Immunoglobulin offers passive immunity and disease protection. Added to the animal feed, the whey protein concentrates have been proven effective in calves and pigs. Strong immunization increases the activity of specific Ig activity for some bacterial antigens.

Casein glycomacropeptide is a protein known to control intestinal microflora. The oligosaccharide of this protein may be its most active component.

Whey and whey permeate (ultra-filtered whey) have been turned into a "bacteriocin-rich dairy ingredient" reported Ahmed E. Yousef, in the Department of Food Sciences and Technology at Ohio State University in Columbus. Bacteriocins are tiny proteins that form when whey and whey permeate are fermented by lactic acid. At least twenty bacteriocins have been identified as effective agents that combat three major pathogens: *Staphylococcus aureus*, *Listeria monocytogenes*, and *Clostridium botulinum.*

Bacteriocins specialize. Each type is effective against only a few types of pathogens. Yousef and his colleagues attempted to custom-design bacteria to produce large amounts of specialized bacteriocins that fight specific pathogens for each type of food that is vulnerable to them.

To produce the bacteriocins, Yousef's team pumped whey or whey permeate, along with selected lactic acid bacteria strains, into a cylindrical bioreactor. The bacteria fermented the liquid and produced lactic acid and bacteriocins.

Whey proteins are separated from casein, the major protein in milk, by isoelectric precipitation or by the action of rennet in cheese production. Whey protein isolate contains about 42 percent protein. The protein efficiency ratio (PER), a formerly used method, found whey protein to have one of the highest biological values. It compared favorably to other protein sources such as egg, milk, beef, soy, and casein. A newer method of measurement that has replaced PER is the protein digestibility-corrected amino acid score (PDCAAS). It, too, ranks whey protein as one of the best protein sources. The level of essential amino acids in whey protein exceeds all other protein sources mentioned above, and comprises about 60 percent of whey's total protein content.

Animal studies with total whey protein have shown beneficial effects on chemically induced cancer, stimulation of the immune system, and increased lifespan. Other animal studies have shown that whey proteins were able to lower low-density lipoprotein (LDL) cholesterol, and promote the release of cholesystokin, an appetite-suppressing hormone.

Whey may be effective against breast cancer. In test-tube experiments, whey inhibited the growth of breast cancer cells.

Whey Protein Hydrolysate

Whey protein consumption may reduce blood pressure. In studies reported in 2000, researchers at the Hypertension Research Institute at Laval University in Quebec, Canada, in collaboration with Davisco Foods International in Eden Prairie, Minnesota, fed whey protein hydrolysate to rats prone to hypertension. The rats' arterial blood pressure was reduced within one to seven hours after they ingested the whey.

Subsequent to this research, hydrolyzed whey protein isolates were found to lower blood pressure in humans, too.

A clinical study reported in 2002, conducted at the Minnesota Medical School in Minneapolis, in collaboration with Davisco Foods, enrolled thirty unmedicated, nonsmoking, borderline hypertensive men and women. One group was given hydrolyzed whey protein isolate in a drink, and the other group (the control) was given an untreated drink. The groups were instructed to consume the drinks daily for six weeks, while maintaining their normal healthy lifestyle habits. After only one week of treatment, the group given the whey drink showed a significant drop both in systolic and diastolic blood pressures. Throughout the six weeks, the group sustained the drop. The untreated group did not experience any drop in blood pressure.

A patented modified whey protein was found to prevent cancer in some laboratory rats. A team of Agricultural Research Service (ARS)– funded investigators, led by neuroendocrinologist and nutritionist Thomas M. Badger, at Arkansas Children's Nutritional Center in Little Rock, studied female Sprague Dawley rats (a strain frequently used in experiments). The animals were fed for three years a diet containing either casein or processed whey protein. At the completion of the study, Badger reported the results. "One hundred percent of the rats fed the casein diet developed mammary tumors, but only about 50 percent of the whey-fed rats developed tumors. In addition, it took longer for the mammary tumors to develop in the whey-fed rats, and they had fewer tumors."

A study in the Netherlands found that whey hydrolysate was useful for colicky infants. The subjects were forty-three infants who, within one week, would cry for more than three hours daily during at least three days during the week. Otherwise, the infants were healthy. All had been fed on standard cow's milk formulas. For a week, half of the infants were switched to a formula made with whey hydrolysate. The other half (the control) continued to consume their regular formulas. All of the children cried less during the week, but the crying decreased an average of one hundred and eleven minutes for the whey-consuming group, compared to a drop of only thirty-four minutes for the control group. The study was reported in *Pediatrics* (Dec 2000).

A type of whey protein, lactoperoxidase, is an enzyme in milk. It has antimicrobial properties that make it potentially useful as an addition to toothpastes and chewing gums.

Glycomacropeptide (GMP)

Glycomacropeptide (GMP) is a protein present in whey. It is cleaved from kappa (κ)-casein by the action of rennet during cheesemaking. GMP has been promoted for its antimicrobial and antitoxic activity, bifidogenic properties, and effects on satiety. GMP contains no phenylalanine, which makes it a suitable protein source for individuals who are phenylketonurics. GMP is potentially useful for infant formulas, dental products, chewing gums, and special dietary foods.

Alpha-lactalbumin

Alpha-lactalbumin is a bioactive whey protein. Studies showed that it boosts the immune system and possesses anticarcinogenic properties. Sometimes it is added to infant-feeding formulas to manufacture products that more closely approximate breastmilk.

Other whey proteins include immunoglobulin. It promotes intestinal health.

Many of these ascribed health benefits are due to the probiotic components in whey. Now, let's examine them individually.

PROBIOTICS IN LACTOFERRIN

Lactoferrin is a naturally occurring iron-binding protein found in all mammal milk. It is the most abundant protein in human colostrum.

Lactoferrin influences the intestinal flora composition in the infant and in the development of a healthy and efficiently functioning immune system. Lactoferrin is involved in biochemical processes in lymphocytes, white blood cells formed in the lymphatic tissues. The white blood cells help ward off infections.

Lactoferrin is involved in iron metabolism, an important factor in the body's defense system against microbial infections. In order to grow and multiply, most bacteria require iron. By binding iron, lactoferrin deprives the bacteria of their needed iron.

In the breastfed infant, lactoferrin can boost immune activity and suppress inflammation. Lactoferrin fights pathogenic viruses, bacteria, and fungi. Even after lactoferrin is broken down in the gut, its fragments continue to fight urinary tract infective agents while they are being voided from the body.

Because lactoferrin lowers the immune system's inflammatory overreactions, this milk protein may be useful against arthritis, multiple sclerosis, and septic shock. In 1998, researchers treated piglets with lactoferrin before intentionally inducing septic shock in the animals. Lactoferrin reduced mortality in the treated piglets to less than one-fourth of the mortality suffered by the untreated animals.

In another experiment, reported in 2001, researchers treated rats with lactoferrin before intentionally induced septic shock. The treated rats showed dramatically reduced concentrations of toxins in their blood.

Lactoferrin is marketed in Asian countries for use in infant-feeding formulas so that the products resemble breastmilk more closely. Cow's milk is the source of commercial lactoferrin. Only about 90 milligrams (mg) per liter (L) of lactoferrin is present in cow's milk, compared to about 1,600 mg/L in human milk. In addition, the colostrum in human fluid contains about 4,900 mg/L of lactoferrin for the newborn infant.

Whether lactoferrin from cow's milk differs from lactoferrin from human breastmilk seems to depend on the uses of the lactoferrin. The presence of receptors specific for human lactoferrin in the infant's digestive tract suggests that lactoferrin acts as the deliverer of iron into the infant's cells. Thus, it may be that only human lactoferrin can affect iron status. Yet, the lactoferrin that is being used as a food supplement is derived from cow's milk. Meanwhile, a "human identical" lactoferrin compound is being made by use of *Aspergillus* strains. Also, lactoferrin is produced by recombinant DNA in transgenic cows. These products can be broken down into different substances and may react differently in the human system. The lactoferrin derived from cow's milk does not bind to the receptor in humans. Both the *Aspergillus*-derived lactoferrin, and the lactoferrin produced by transgenic cows, do bind to the receptor and deliver iron to human cells. It is moot, however, whether biologically engineered compounds deserve to be regarded as "nature identical."

At the annual meeting of the Institute of Food Technologists in 1997, a symposium was held on "Bioactive Components in Milk." Bo Lönnerdal, a nutritionist from the University of California at Davis, reported at the symposium that lactoferrin binds to lipopolysaccharides (fats attached to sugars), and can bind two iron atoms per molecule. Lactoferrin in human milk is in the unsaturated form. During the first few months of an infant's life, quantities of lactoferrin pass through the infant's digestive tract. Lönnerdal recommended that studies be conducted to ensure that the bovine lactoferrin, added to infant foods, and to special medical foods, actually is effective.

In recent years, lactoferrin is manufactured increasingly as a probiotic for use in functional and sports beverages, dietary supplements, and chewing gums.

The activated lactoferrin deprives iron to pathogens on fresh beef surfaces, and prevents the pathogens from growing or surviving. Activated lactoferrin has been shown to be effective against more than thirty pathogens, including virulent ones such as *Escherichia coli* 0157:H7, and certain strains of *Salmonella* and *Listeria*.

PROBIOTICS IN PEPTIDES

Peptides are related to proteins insofar as both contain amino acids. Many bioactive peptides have been identified in milk, as casein or whey-protein precursors. The peptides derived from casein are casomorphins. Some are opioid antagonists that bond to opioid receptors. They exhibit morphine-like qualities. Others, derived from lactoferrin or κ-casein, suppress the agonist activity of enkephalins (closely related peptides with opiate qualities, and found in the brain, spinal cord, and other parts of the body) and affect the smooth muscles. These bioactive peptides also function as carriers of minerals in the body. The glycomacropeptides form during cheesemaking, from the reaction of chymosin (a protein-digesting enzyme) with κ-casein. Whey consists of 15 to 20 percent glycomacropeptides.

PROBIOTICS IN MILKFAT

The milkfat in milk also contains some components that are probiotic agents. "Milkfat is the most complex system known," remarked Joseph O'Donnell, director of the California Dairy Research Foundation in Davis. O'Donnell reported that milkfat contains potential anticarcinogenic components, including conjugated linoleic acid (CLA), sphingomyelin, butyric acid, and other fats.

CLA is a naturally occurring fatty acid found mainly in the fat of dairy products and meats such as beef and lamb. CLA consists of one or more positional and geometric isomers of linoleic acid (*cis*-9, *cis*-12-octa-decadienoic acid). CLA's conjugated double bonds are usually at position 9, 11, or 10 and 12, with each double bond either in the *cis* or *trans* configuration. (The *trans* configuration puzzles the public, which has been told that *trans* fatty acids are bad and should be avoided. CLA is a "good" *trans* fat, unlike *trans* fats that result from the hydrogenation process.)

CLA has been found to have numerous beneficial health effects. It acts as an antioxidant. It helps maintain a healthy heart and veins, and healthy cholesterol and triglyceride levels. It combats atherosclerosis. It encourages the buildup of muscles and helps prevent weight gain. Preschoolers who have an optimal intake of CLA in the diet are less likely to suffer from asthma when they are older. But, perhaps the most impressive feature, is that CLA is the only known fatty acid to have strong anticarcinogenic properties. CLA has been shown to inhibit the growth of a variety of human tumor cells, including cancer cells of the skin, colon, heart, and lung. Also, animal studies showed that CLA prevents the spread of cancer.

Australian studies published by the American Society for Nutritional Sciences showed that CLA inhibited the proliferation of malignant melanomas as well as colorectal, breast, and lung cancer cell lines. In mouse studies, CLA reduced the incidence of chemically induced epidermal tumors and forestomach neoplasia (the formation of new tissue). In rat studies, CLA reduced the incidence of aberrant crypt foci, which are precancerous.

Unfortunately, less than optimal amounts of CLA are consumed by Americans. There are several reasons: changes in agricultural practices, changes in dietary choices, and mixed messages from governmental agencies.

Cud-chewing animals (ruminants such as cows) have bacteria that convert linoleic acid into CLA. However, the CLA content of the milkfat of cows and the CLA content of the fat in beef has declined steadily as the animals have been switched from grass grazing in pastures to grain feeding in feedlots. These changed practices yield greater volumes of milk from cows, and quicker weight gain in beef animals, at the expense of CLA and other beneficial components. Also, the feeding of dry hay in wintertime offers no CLA in the feed.

Due to changes in dietary choices, most Americans fail to consume adequate amounts of CLA. Many people select low- or non-fat milk and other dairy products, and avoid butter and cream. Many people also foolishly shun red meats or limit their intake and discard any visible fat in the meat.

Governmental agencies have been sending mixed messages. They have recommended reduction of saturated fats (sources of CLA) and have encouraged the substitution of vegetable oils (lacking in CLA). They have labeled trans fats as "bad" and fail to acknowledge that CLA, a trans fat, is beneficial. The FDA had wrestled with this problem, when it formulated a regulation mandating food manufacturers to indicate the trans fats in food products. The agency considered exempting CLA from the regulations, but decided it would be too confusing for the public.

Beef and lamb fat also contain another fatty acid, palmitoleic acid. This substance protects humans from viruses and other pathogens.

These various findings should arouse some curiosity in scientists. The time has come to reexamine the commonly held belief that butter, cream, whole milk, and animal fats should be limited or avoided.

PROBIOTICS IN SPHINGOLIPIDS

Sphingolipids are fat membranes consisting of sphingomyelin and glycosphingolipids. Sphingomyelin is a phospholipid located in the outer leaflet of the plasma membrane of most mammalian cells. In cow's milk, phospholipids represent from 0.2 to 1.0 grams per 100 grams of total fat. They are associated with the milkfat globule. Glycosphingolipids are sugars attached to sphingolipids. The sphingolipids have lipid backbones that serve as secondary messengers in regulating cell activity, including growth, differentiation, and apotosis (cell death). Sphingomyelin is hydrolyzed (broken down by means of water) to the lipid backbone during normal digestion. E. M. Schmelz from Emory University in Atlanta, Georgia, found that sphingomyelin suppressed a number of early markers of colonic cancer. The amount of sphingomyelin used in the studies was about the same amount that would be present in dairy products.

PROBIOTICS IN BUTYRIC ACID

Butyric acid, another milk component, has been shown to regulate apoto-sis by inhibiting uncontrolled proliferation of cells and supporting nor-mal cell death in a number of types of cancer cells. J. B. German at the University of California at Davis, reported research on the role of butyric acid as the result of fermenting fiber in the digestive system, as well as its role as an anticancer agent. Butyric acid was found to eliminate cancer cells from the tissues that line the lower intestine. Apparently, butyric acid increases the process of programmed cell death in cancer cells, but not in healthy tissue. The use of vegetable-based fiber as a starting mate-rial to develop butyric acid in these studies is somewhat puzzling. The natural source of butyric acid is milkfat.

Bioactive Probiotic Colostrum: A Special Mammary Fluid

Colostrum is a thick fluid produced in all female mammals to feed their newly born offspring before the actual milk production begins. Breastfed infants derive probiotics from colostrum, denied to formula-fed ones. Similarly, newborn calves allowed to ingest bovine colostrum from their mothers derive probiotic benefits; calves fed formulas are denied probiotic benefits. Formula feeding for human infants and for calves can only approximate the complex compositions of species-specific mammalian milks. Supplementation of formulas with bovine colostrum for human infants denies a birthright to optimal nourishment.

PROBIOTICS IN COLOSTRUM

Colostrum is produced in a woman's breast during the first day or two after she has given birth. Over time, the benefits of colostrum have come to be better recognized, not only for the newly born infant, but also as a medical adjuvant.

Colostrum contains immune factors such as a broad spectrum of antibodies, intended to protect the infant against pathogenic bacteria, viruses, and parasites. Colostrum also contains growth factors such as the growth hormone IGF-1 that promotes the repair and regeneration of bone, muscle, skin, nerves, tissues, and cartilage.

It is thought that colostrum may be useful as a probiotic supplement to treat autoimmune conditions, such as rheumatoid arthritis, by balancing an overactive immune system that attacks healthy cells. Also, some investigators theorize that because colostrum has antioxidant properties and rejuvenating power of the immune system and growth factors, it may be useful in retarding diseases of aging.

In 1962, Dr. Albert Sabin developed the polio vaccine from antibodies isolated from colostrum. Since then, studies showed that colostrum has an abundance of vitamins and minerals, as well as antioxidants. In analysis, colostrum was found to contain more than twenty times the amount of vitamin B_{12} than contained in regular milk. This vitamin is an immune booster.

A study reported in *Pediatric Infectious Disease* (Sarker, 1998) found that bovine colostrum was an effective treatment for acute rotavirus diarrhea in infants.

A modest study reported in *Bone Marrow Transplantation* (Tollemar, 1999) found that bovine colostrum drastically reduced fungal infections in seven out of ten bone marrow transplant recipients. Ordinarily, such patients have a high risk of infection and death.

Rat studies, reported in *Gut* (Playford, 1999), showed that colostrum reduced gastrointestinal impairment such as ulcers caused by nonsteroidal anti-inflammatory drugs (NSAIDs) by 60 percent. Frequently, NSAIDs are used for long time periods by individuals with autoimmune diseases.

The natural immune components (antibodies) in colostrum are proteins produced by white blood cells and secreted into the colostrum. Also present in colostrum are nonspecific immune substances, lactoferrin and lactoperoxidase.

BIOACTIVE COMPONENTS IN COLOSTRUM

There are impressive numbers of bioactive components in colostrum that act as probiotics. Here are some of the components and their roles.

- Immunoglobulin IgA, IgD, IgE, IgG, and IgM help combat pathogens and neutralize toxins.

- Lactoferrin has antimicrobial properties.

- Proline-rich polypeptides (PRPs) are hormones that stimulate immunity and regulate the thymus gland.

- Leukocyte blood cells stimulate interferon production, inhibit viral penetration of cell walls, and slow viral reproduction.

- Lactoperoxidase thiocyanate, peroxidase, and xanthine release hydrogen peroxide and destroy pathogens.

- Cytokines intensify immune response and boost T-cell activity, and control cell-to-cell communications.

- Glycoproteins and trypsin inhibitors protect immune and growth factors in colostrum from being destroyed in the GI tract, as well as preventing *Helicobacter pylori* from attaching to the stomach wall.

- Lymphokines are hormone-like peptides that regulate immune system responses.

- Oligopolysaccharides and glycoconjugate saccharides bind to pathogens such as *Streptococcus, Salmonella, Cryptosporidia, Giardia, Entamoeba, Shigella, Clostridium difficile, Vibrio cholera, Escherichia* toxin A and B, and cholera, and prevent their attachment to the intestinal mucosa.

- Additional immune factors in colostrum include orotic acid, secretory IgA cells, IgA specific helper cells.

COLOSTRUM: AVAILABLE FOR ALL AGES

Increasingly, bovine colostrum is being added to functional foods, as well as to commonly sold foods such as smoothies, yogurts, ice creams, fruit and vegetable juice beverages, and snack foods.

Bovine colostrum is available, too, as probiotic supplements, in capsule, tablet, powder, and liquid forms. These products vary in quality. Ellen Cutler, author of *Winning the War Against Immune Disorders* (Thomson Learning, 1998), recommends that consumers seek colostrum supplements produced in New Zealand, because of the strict farming standards in that country.

Colostrum may cause bloating. Rare and temporary side effects include itching, headaches, and muscle aches. If such supplements are taken late in the day, they may cause temporary insomnia. Colostrum is best absorbed if it is taken with at least eight ounces of water.

Main Sources

Introduction

Farnsworth, ER. "The Beneficial Health Effects of Fermented Foods: Potential Probiotics Around the World." *J Nutraceut Function Med Fd,* Vol 4, 2004, 93–117

"Food Quackery." *Consumers All.* USDA Yearbook, 1965, 414

Fuller, R. "Probiotics in Man and Animals." *J Appl Bacteriol,* Vol 66, 1989, 365–378

Guidelines for the Evaluation of Probiotics in Food. Report of a Joint FAO/WHO Working Group. London, Ontario, Can: 2002

Havenaar, R & JHJ Huis in't Veld. "Probiotics: A General View" in *The Lactic Acid Bacteria in Health & Disease,* Vol 1, BJB Wood, ed, London, Eng: Elsevier Appl Sci, 1992

Lee, YK & S Salminen. "The Coming of Age of Probiotics." *Trends Fd Sci Technol,* Vol 6, 1999, 241–244

Marx, J. "Puzzling Out the Pains in the Gut." *Sci,* Vol 315, Jan 5, 2007, 33–35

"New Bacterial Defense Against Phage Invaders Identified." *Sci,* Mar 23, 2007, 1650–1651

Parker, RB. "Probiotics, the Other Half of the Antibiotic Story." *Anim Nutr Health,* Vol 29, 1974, 48

Reuter, G. "Present & Future Probiotics in Germany & in Central Europe." *Biosci Microflora,* Vol 16, 1997, 43–51

Wildman, RE, ed. *Handbook of Nutraceuticals & Functional Foods.* 2nd ed. Boca Raton, Fl: CRC Press, 346–347

Wood, BJB, ed. *The Lactic Acid Bacteria in Health & Disease.* Vol l, London, Eng: Elsevier Appl Sci, 1992

Chapter 1

Brudnak, MA. *The Probiotic Solution.* St. Paul, MN: Dragon Door Publ, 2003

Deis, RC. "Opportunities for Heart-Healthy Food." *Fd Prod Design*, Feb 2007, 63–75

"Diving into Dairy Development." *Prep Fds*, Jan 2007, 113–122

Fuller, R. "Probiotics in Man and Animals." *J Appl Bacteriol*, Vol 66, 1989, 365–378

—— "Probiotics for Farm Animals" in *Probiotic: A Critical Review*. GW Tannock, ed. Wymondham UK: Horizon Sci Press, 1998, 15–22

"Functional Dairy: On Top and Growing—Business Strategies, Healthy Foods." *Functional Fds Nutraceut*, May 2007, 22; 24

Gerdes, S. "Yogurt: Enhancing a Superfood." *Fd Prod Design*, Mar 2007, 68–80

Gill, HS & F Guarnet. "Probiotics and Human Health: A Clinical Perspective." *Postgrad Med J*, Vol 80, No 947, 2004, 516–526

Guarmer, F & GJ Schaafsma. "Probiotics." *Internatl J Fd Microbiol*, Vol 39, 2000, 237–238

Guidelines for the Evaluation of Probiotics in Food. FAO/WHO, London, Ontario, Can, 2002

Kimbrell, W et al. "Mass Appeal." *Dairy Fds*, Vol 91, No 2, Feb 1990, 43–47; 50–65

Lee, YK, K Nomoto, S Saiminen & SI Gorbach. *Handbook of Probiotics*. NY: John Wiley & Sons, 1999

O'Donnell, CD. "Buying into Bioactives." *Prep Fds Nutra Sols*, Mar 2004, NS 9

"Probing Probiotics." *Prep Fds*, Jan 2007, 9

"Probiotics' Flourishing Future." *Functional Fds Nutraceut*, Dec 2005, 28–31

Reid, G & J Hammond. "Probiotics: Some Evidence of Their Effectiveness." *Can Fam Phy*, Vol 51, 2005, 1487–1493

Rice, J. "Probiotics & Prebiotics for Healthful Benefits." *Fd Prod Design*, July 2002, 61–71

Roberts, Jr. WA. "Forecasting Food's Future." *Prep Fds*, Jan 2007, 27

Salminen, SJ, M Gueimonds & E Isolauri. "Probiotics That Modify Disease Risk." *J Nutr*, Vol 135, No 5, 2005, 1294–1298

Townsend, J. "Probiotics for the Future." *Functional Fds Nutraceut*, Jan 2007, 48

Chapter 2

Kiple, KF & KC Ornelas. *The Cambridge World History of Food*. NY: Cambridge University Press, 2000

Tannahill, R. *Food in History*. NY: Stein & Day, 1973

Chapter 3

Beuchat, LR. "Application of Biotechnology to Indigenous Fermented Foods." *Fd Tech*, Jan 1995, 97–99

Campbett-Pratt, G. *Fermented Foods of the World: A Dictionary and Guide*. London, Eng: Butterworths, 1987

Hesseltine, CW. "Microbiology of Oriental Fermented Foods." *Ann Rev Microb*, Vol 37, 1983, 575–601

Hesseltine, CW & HL Wang. "Indigenous Fermented Food of Non-Western Origin." *Mycologia Memori*, No 11, Berlin, Ger: J Cramer, 1986

Steinkraus, KH. *Handbook of Indigenous Fermented Foods*. NY: Marcel Dekker, 1983

Chapter 4

"Ingredients For and From Fermentation." *Fd Tech*, Dec 1993, 93–98

McBean, LD. "Emerging Dietary Benefits of Dairy Foods." *Nutr Today*, Vol 34, No 1, 1999, 47–53

Robinson, RK, ed. *Therapeutic Properties of Fermented Milks*. NY: Elsevier Appl Sci, 1991

Spiller, Cheryl Solomon. "Fermented Food." *Natural Health*, Apr 2000, 147

Toops, Diane. "Yogurt in All Its Forms." *Fd Proc*, June 2004, 38–39

Chapter 5

Metchnikoff, I. *The Prolongation of Life*. NY: GP Putnam's Sons, 1908

Rosell, JM. "Yoghourt & Kefir in the Relation to Health & Therapeutics." *Can Med Assoc J*, Vol 26, 1932, 34–45

Seneca, H et al. "Bacterial Properties of Yogurt." *Am Practition Digest Treat*, Vol 12, Dec 1950

Chapter 6

Constipation

Marteau, P et al. "*Bifidobacterium animalis* Strain DN-173 010 Shortens the Colonic Transit Time in Healthy Women: A Double-Blind, Randomized Controlled Study." *Aliment Pharmacol Ther*, Vol 16, 2002, 587–598

Meance, S et al. "A Fermented Milk with *Bifidobacterium* Probiotic Strain DN-173-010 Shortened Oro-Fecal Gut Transit Time in Elderly." *Microbiol Ecol Health Dis*, Vol 13, 2001, 217–222

Crohn's Disease

Borruel, N et al. "Increased Mucosal Tumor Necrosis Factor Alpha Production in Crohn's Disease Can Be Downrated *Ex vivo* by Probiotic Bacteria." *Gut*, Vol 51, No 5, Nov 2002, 659–664

Malin, M et al. "Promotion of IgA Immune Response in Patients with Crohn's Disease by Oral Bacteriotherapy with *Lactobacillus* GG." *Ann Nutr Metabol*, Vol 40, 1996, 137–145

Diarrhea

Bodilis, JY. "Controlled Clinical Trial of Lacteol Fort Compared with a Placebo & Reference Drug in the Treatment of Acute Diarrhea in the Adult." *Med Actuelle*, Vol 10, 1983, 232–235

Chauviére, G et al. "Adhesion of Human *Lactobacillus acidophilus* Strain LB to Human Enterocyte-like Caco-2 Cells." *J Gen Microb*, Vol 138, 1992, 1689–1696

Clements, ML et al. "*Lactobacillus* Prophylaxis for Diarrhea Due to Enterotoxigenic *Escherichia coli*." *Antimicrob Agents Chemother*, Vol 20, 1981, 104–108

Gotz, V et al. "Prophylaxis Against Ampillin-Associated Diarrhea with a *Lactobacillus* Preparation." *Am J Hosp Pharm*, Vol 36, 1979, 754–757

Kaila, M et al. "Enhancement of the Circulating Antibody Secreting Cell Response in Human Diarrhea by a Human *Lactobacillus* Strain." *Pediat Res*, Vol 32, 1992, 141–144

Pedone, CA et al. "Multicentric Study of the Effect of Milk Fermented by *Lactobacillus casei* in the Incidence of Diarrhea." *Internatl J Clin Pract*, Vol 54, 2000, 568–571

Pereg, D et al. "The Effect of Fermented Yogurt on the Prevention of Diarrhea in a Healthy Adult Population." *Am J Infect Control*, Vol 33, 2005, 122–125

Sanders, ME. "Healthful Attributes of Bacteria in Yogurt." *Contemp Nutr*, Vol 18, No 5, 1993, 1

Sullivan, PB. "Nutritional Management of Acute Diarrhea." *Nutr*, Vol 14, 1998, 758–762

Wunderlich, PF et al. "Double-Blind Report on the Efficacy of Lactic Acid-Producing *Enterococcus* SF68 in the Prevention of Antibiotic-Associated Diarrhoea & in the Treatment of Active Diarrhoea." *J Int Med Res*, Vol 17, 1989, 833–838

Gastrointestinal Tract

Anthony, M. "Digestive Health's New Phase." *Fd Proc Wellness Fds*, Aug 2006, 22

Arrigoni, E et al. "Tolerance & Absorption of Lactose from Milk & Yogurt during Short-Bowel Syndrome in Humans."*Am J Clin Nutr,* Vol 60, 1994, 926–929

Axelsson, LT et al. "Production of a Broad-Spectrum Antimicrobial Substance by *Lactobacillus reuteri.*" *Microb Ecol Health Dis,* Vol 2, 1989, 131–136

Bengmark, S. "Ecological Control of the Gastrointestinal Tract: The Role of Probiotic Flora." *Gut,* Vol 42, 1998, 2–7

Benno, Y et al. "The Intestinal Microflora of Infants: Composition of Fecal Flora in Breast-Fed & Bottle-Fed Infants." *Microbiol Immunol,* Vol 28, 1984, 975–986

Bernet, MF et al. "*Lactobacillus acidophilus* LA Binds to Human Intestinal Cell Lines & Inhibits Cell Attachment & Cell Invasion by Enterovirulent Bacteria." *Gut,* Vol 35, 1994, 483–489

Biller, JA et al. "Treatment of Recurrent *Clostridium difficile* Colitis with *Lactobacillus* GG." *J Pediat Gastroenterol Nutr,* Vol 21, 1995, 224–226

Bouhnik, Y et al. "Fecal Recovery in Human of Viable *Bifidobacterium* sp Ingested in Fermented Milk." Vol 102, 1992, 875–878

Buchanan, RL & MP Doyle. "Foodborne Disease Significance of *Escherichia coli* 0157:H7 and Other Enterohemorrhagic *E. coli.* A Scientific Status Summary by the Institute of Food Technology's Expert Panel on Food Safety & Nutrition." *Fd Tech,* Vol 51, No 10, 1997, 69–76

Coconnier, MH et al. "Inhibition of Adhesion on Enteroinvasive Pathogens to Human Intestinal Caco-2 Cells by *Lactobacillus acidophilus* Strain LB Decreases Bacterial Invasion." *FEMS Microbiol Lett,* Vol 110, 1993, 299–306

Colombel, JF et al. "Yoghurt with *Bifidobacterium longum* Reduced Erythromycin-Induced Gastrointestinal Effect." *Lancet* II, 1987, 43

Fuller, R. "Probiotics in Human Medicine." *Gut,* Vol 32, 1991, 439–442

Goldin, BR & SL Gorbach. "The Effect of Milk & *Lactobacillus* Feeding on Human Intestinal Bacterial Enzyme Activity." *Am J Clin Nutr,* 39, 1984, 756–761

—— et al. "Survival of *Lactobacillus* Species (Strain GG) in the Human Gastrointestinal Tract." *Dig Dis Sci,* Vol 37, 1992, 121–128

Gorbach, SI et al. "Successful Treatment of Relapsing *Clostridium difficile* with *Lactobacillus* GG."*J Pediat Gastroenterol, Lancet* II, 1987, 1519

Gorman, J. "Aliens Inside Us: A (Mostly) Friendly Bacterial Nation." *NY Times,* Apr 1, 2003, D3

Hentges, DJ. "Gut Flora and Disease Resistance" in *Probiotics: The Scientific Basis.* R Fuller, ed., London, Eng: Chapman & Hall, 1992

Hill, MJ. "Diet & the Human Intestinal Bacterial Flora." *Cancer Res,* Vol 41, 1981, 3778–3780

Holzapfel, TH et al. "Overview of Gut Flora & Probiotics." *Internatl J Fd Microbiol,* Vol 41, 1998, 85–101

Hunter, BT, *Food & Your Health.* North Bergen, NJ: Basic Health Publications, 2003, 312–360

Lidbeck, A et al. " Impact of *Lactobacillus acidophilus* Supplements on the Human Oropharyngeal & Intestinal Microflora." *Scand J Infect Dis,* Vol 19, 1987, 531–537

Mitsuoka, T. "Intestinal Flora & Aging." *Nutr Rev,* Vol 50, No 12, Dec 1992, 438–446

Orrhage, K et al. "Effects of Supplements of *Bifidobacterium longum* & *Lactobacillus acidophilus* on the Intestinal Microbiota during Administration of Clindamycin." *Microb Ecol Health Disease,* Vol 7, 1994, 17–25

"Probiotics." Scientific Status Summary. Expert Panel on Food Safety & Nutrition. *Fd Tech,* Vol 53, No 1, Nov 1999, 67–77

Rambaud, JC et al. "Manipulation of the Human Gut Microflora." *Proc Nutr Soc,* 1993, 357–366

Rolfe, D. "Probiotics: Prospect for Use in *Clostridum difficile*-associated Intestinal Disease," in *Probiotics: Prospects of Use in Opportunistic Infections,* R Fuller, PJ Heidt, V Rusch, DVD Waaiki, eds. Herborn, Ger: Inst for Microecol, 1995, 47–66

Rubalterri, FF et al. "Intestinal Flora in Breast & Bottle-Fed Infants." *J Pediat Med,* Vol 26, 1998, 186–189

Teitelbaum, JE & WA Walker. "Nutritional Impact of Pre- & Probiotics as Protective Gastrointestinal Organisms." *Ann Rev Nutr,* Vol 22, 2002, 107–138

Vanderbergh, PA. "Lactic Acid Bacteria, Their Metabolic Products, & Interference with Microbial Growth." *FEMS Microbiol Rev,* Vol 12, 1993, 221–238

Helicobacter pylori

Aiba, Y et al. "Lactic Acid-Mediated Suppression of *Helicobacter pylori* by the Oral Administration of *Lactobacillus pylori* & *Lactobacillus salivarius* as a Probiotic in a Gnotobiotic Murine Model." *Am J Gastroenterol,* Vol 93, 1998, 2097–2101

Kabir, AM et al. "Prevention of *Helicobacter pylori* Infection by *Lactobacilli* in a Gnotobiotic Murine Model." *Gut,* Vol 41, 1997, 49–56

Marshall, BJ. "*Helicobacter pylori.*" *Am J Gastroenterol,* Vol 89, Suppl, 1994, S116–S128

Mindolo, PD et al. "In Vitro Inhibition of *Helicobacter pylori* NCTC 11637 by Organic Acids & Lactic Acid Bacteria, *J Appl Bacteriol,* Vol 79, 1995, 475–479

Inflammatory Bowel Disease

Chermesh, I & R Eliakim. "Probiotics: Scope & Promise in Inflammatory Bowel Disease." *Israel Med Assoc J*, Vol 4, No 5, May 2002, 353–356

Targan, R & F Shanahan, *Inflammatory Bowel Disease from Bench to Bedside*. Baltimore, MD: Williams & Wilkins, 1994

Irritable Bowel Syndrome

Halpern, GH et al. "Treatment of Irritable Bowel Syndrome with Lacteol Fort: A Randomized, Double-Blind Cross-Over Trial." *Am J Gastroenterol*, Vol 91, 1996, 1579–1585

Infant Diarrhea

Bellomo, G et al. "A Controlled Double-Blinded Study of SF68 Strain as a New Biological Preparation for the Treatment of Diarrhea in Pediatrics." *Curr Therap Res,* Vol 28, 1980, 927–936

Bhatnagar, S et al. "Efficacy of Milk Versus Yogurt Offered as Part of a Mixed Diet in Acute Noncholera Diarrhea Amongst Malnourished Children." *J Pediat,* Vol 132, 1998, 999–1003

Boulloche, J et al. "Management of Acute Diarrhoea in Infants & Children: Controlled Study of the Antidiarrhoeal Efficacy of Killed *Acidophilus* (LB Strain)." *Ann Pediat,* Vol 41, 1994, 457–463

Gonzalez, S et al. "Prevention of Infantile Diarrhea by Fermented Milk." *Microbiol Aliments Nutr,* Vol 8, 1997, 349–355

Isolauri, E et al. "A Human *Lactobacillus* Strain (*Lactobacillus casei* sp Strain GG) Promotes Recovery from Acute Diarrhea in Children." *Pediat,* Vol 88, 1991, 90–97

Leary, WE. "Two Healthful Bacteria Are Proved to Ward Off Diarrhea in Infants." *NY Times,* Oct 14, 1994, A29

Pedone, CA et al. "The Effect of Supplementation with Milk Fermented by *Lactobacillus casei* (Strain DN-114-001) on Acute Diarrhea in Children Attending Day Care Centers." *Internatl J Clin Proc,* Vol 53, 1999, 181–184

Szajewska, H et al. "Probiotics in the Prevention of Antibiotic-Associated Diarrhea in Children: A Meta-Analysis of Randomized Controlled Trials." *J Pediat,* Vol 149, Sept 2006, 367–372

Touhami, M et al. "Clinical Consequences of Replacing Milk with Yogurt in Persistent Infantile Diarrhea." *Ann Pediat,* Vol 39, 1992, 79–86

Vanderhouf, JA & RJ Young. "Use of Probiotics in Childhood Gastrointestinal Disorders." *J Pediat Gastroenterol Nutr*, Vol 27, 1988, 323–332

Rotavirus

Friedrich, MJ. "A Bit of Culture for Children: Probiotics May Improve Health & Fight Disease." Medical News & Perspectives. *JAMA*, Vol 284, No 11, Sept 20, 2000, 1365–1366

Isolauri, E et al. "Improved Immunogenicity of Oral Dx RRV Reassortant Rotavirus Vaccine by *Lactobacillus casei* GG." *Vaccine*, Vol 13, 1995, 310–312

Majamaa, H et al. "Lactic Acid Bacteria in the Treatment of Acute Rotavirus Gastroenteritis." *Pediat Gastroenterol Nutr*, Vol 20, No 3, Apr 1995, 333–338

Parashar, UD et al. "Rotavirus." *Emer Infect Dis*, Vol 4, 1998, 561–570

Saavedra, JM et al. "Feeding of *Bifidobacterium bifidum* and *Streptococcus thermophilus* to Infants in Hospitals for Prevention of Diarrhea & Shedding of Rotavirus." *Lancet*, Vol 344, 1994, 1046–1049

Travelers' Diarrhea

"Biopharmaceuticals." *Fd Engineer*, Dec 1989, 58

deDios-Poso-Alano, J et al. "Effect of a *Lactobacilli* Preparation on Traveler's Diarrhea: A Randomized, Double-Blind Clinical Trial." *Gastroenterol*, Vol 74, 1998, 829–830

Elmer, GW. "Biotherapeutic Agents: A Neglected Modality for the Treatment & Prevention of Selected Intestinal & Vaginal Infections." *JAMA*, Vol 275, No 11, Mar 20, 1996, 870–876

Hunter, BT. *Food & Your Health*. North Bergen, NJ: Basic Health Publications, 2003, 330–334

Oksanen, PJ et al. "Prevention of Travelers' Diarrhoea by *Lactobacillus* GG." *Ann Med*, Vol 22, 1990, 53–56

Chapter 7

Archibald, Manada. "Mounting an Immune Defense." *Prep Fds Nutra Sols*, Nov 2003, NS 307

Bocci, V. "The Neglected Organ: Bacterial Flora Has a Critical Immunostimulatory Role." *Perspect Biol Med*, Vol 35, No 2, Winter 1992, 251–260

Chiang, BL et al. "Enhancing Immunity by Dietary Consumption of a Probiotic

Lactic Acid Bacterium (*Bifidobacterium lactis* HN 019) Optimization and Definition of Cellular Immune Response." *Eur J Clin Nutr,* Vol 54, 2000, 848–855

DeSimone, C et al. "The Role of Probiotics in Modulation of the Immune System in Man & in Animals." *Internatl J Immunotherap,* Vol 9, 1993, 23–28

Ezedam, JH van Loveren. "Probiotics' Immunomodulation & Evaluation of Safety & Efficacy." *Nutr Rev,* Vol 64, No 1, 2006, 1–14

Gill, HS. "Stimulation of the Immune System by Lactic Cultures." *Internatl Dairy J,* Vol 8, 1998, 535–544

——— et al. "Enhancement of Immunity in the Elderly by Dietary Supplementation with the Probiotic *Bifidobacterium lactis* HN019." *Am J Clin Nutr,* Vol 74, 2001, 833–839

Gustafsson, BE. "The Physiological Importance of the Colonic Microflora." *Scand J Gastroenterol,* Vol 77, 1982, 117–131

Link-Amster, H et al. "Modulation of a Specific Humoral Immune Response & Changes in Intestinal Flora Mediated through Fermented Milk Intake." *FEMS Immunol Med Microbiol,* Vol 10, 1994, 56–64

McCracken, BJ & HR Gaskins. "Probiotics & the Immune System," in *Probiotics: A Critical Review,* GW Tannock, ed., Norfolk, Eng: Horizon Sci Press, 1999, 85–111

Morimoto, K et al. "Modulation of Natural Killer Cell Activity by Supplementation of Fermented Milk Containing *Lactobacillus casei* in Habitual Smokers." *Prevent Med,* Vol 40, May 2005, 589–601

Perdigón, G & S Alvarez. "Probiotics & the Immune State," in *Probiotics: The Scientific Basis,* R Fuller, ed., London, Eng: Chapman & Hall, 1992, 145–179

——— et al. "Immune System Stimulation by Probiotics." *J Dairy Sci,* Vol 78, 1995, 1597–1606

Sanders, ME. "Healthful Attributes of Bacteria in Yogurt." *Contemp Nutr,* Vol 18, No 5, 1993, 1

Schultz, M et al. "Immunomodulatory Consequences of Oral Administration of *Lactobacillus rhamnosus* Strain GG in Healthy Volunteers." *J Dairy Res,* Vol 70, No 2, May 2003, 165–173

Spanhaak, S et al. "The Effect of Consumption of Milk Fermented by *Lactobacillus casei* Strain *Shirota* on the Intestinal Microflora & Immune Parameters in Humans." *Eur J Clin Nutr,* Vol 52, 1998, 907

Targan, SR et al. "Immunologic Mechanisms in Intestinal Diseases." *Ann Intern Med,* Vol 106, 1987, 855–870

Trapp, CL et al. "The Influence of Chronic Yogurt Consumption on Populations of Young & Elderly Adults." *J Immunother,* Vol 9, 1993, 53–64

Wheeler, JG. "Immune & Clinical Impact of *Lactobacillus acidophilus* on Asthma." *Ann Allerg Asthma Immunol,* Vol 19, 1997, 229–233

—— et al. "Impact of Dietary Yogurt on Immune Function." *Am J Med Sci,* Vol 313, 1997, 120–123

"Yogurt Found Immunogenic." *Med Trib,* Apr 23, 1991, 20

Chapter 8

Aldinucci, C et al. "Effects of Dietary Yoghurt on Immunological & Clinical Parameters of Rhinopathic Patients." *Eur J Clin Nutr,* Vol 56, Dec 2002, 1155–1161

Beaudette, T & R Strickland. *Food Sensitivity.* Chicago, IL: Am Diet Assoc, 1985

——. *Gluten Intolerance.* Chicago, IL: Am Diet Assoc, 1985

——. *Lactose Intolerance.* Chicago, IL: Am Diet Assoc, 1959

Coca, AF. *The Pulse Test.* NY: Arc Bks, 1959

Del Giudice, M & M Del Guido. "The Role of Probiotics in the Clinical Management of Food Allergy & Atopic Dermatitis." *J Clin Gastroenterol,* Vol 38, July 2004, S84–S85

Fisher, M. *Enjoy Nutritious Variety.* Evanston, IL: Nutr for Optimal Health Assoc, 1980

Friedrich, MJ. "A Bit of Culture for Children: Probiotics May Improve Health & Fight Disease." Medical News and Perspectives." *JAMA,* Vol 284, No 11, Sept 20, 2000, 1365–1366

Garvie, EI et al. "The Effects of Yogurt on Some Components of the Gut Microflora & in the Metabolism of Lactose in the Rat." *J Appl Bacteriol,* Vol 56, 1984, 237–245

Gilliland, SE & HS Kim. "Effect of Viable Starter Culture Bacteria in Yogurt on Lactose Utilization in Humans." *J Dairy Sci,* Vol 67, 1994, 1–6

Hatakka, K et al. "Effect of Long-term Consumption of Probiotic Milk on Infections in Children Attending Day Care Centers: Double-Blind, Randomized Trial." *JAMA* abstract, July 25, 2001, 399

Isolauri, E et al. "*Lactobacillus casei* Strain GG Reverses Increased Intestinal Permeability Induced by Cow Milk in Suckling Rats." *Gastroenterol,* Vol 105, 1993, 1643–1650

Kolars, JC et al. "Yogurt: An Autodigesting Source of Lactose." *N Engl J Med,* Vol 310, 1984, 1–3

Lerebours, E et al. "Yogurt & Fermented-Then-Pasteurized Milk: Effects on Short-

Term & Long-Term Ingestion on Lactose Absorption & Mucosal Lactase Activity in Lactase-Deficient Subjects." *Am J Clin Nutr,* Vol 49, 1989, 823–827

Majamaa, H & E Isolauri. "Probiotics: A Novel Approach in the Management of Food Allergy." *J Allergy Clin Immunol,* Vol 99, No 2, Feb 1997, 179–185

Pelto, L et al. "*Lactobacillus* GG Modulates Milk-Induced Immuno-Inflammatory Response in Milk Hypersensitive Adults." *Nutr Today,* Vol 31, Suppl, 1996, 45S–46S

Pochart, P et al. "Viable Starter Culture, Beta Galactosidase Activity, & Lactose in Duodenum after Yogurt Ingestion in Lactase-Deficient Humans." *Am J Clin Nutr,* Vol 49, 1989, 828–831

Rosenfeldt, V et al. "Effect of Probiotics on Gastrointestinal Symptoms & Small Intestinal Permeability in Children with Atopic Dermatitis." *J Pediat,* Vol 145, Nov 2004, 612–616

Sanders, ME. "Healthful Attributes of Bacteria in Yogurt." *Contemp Nutr,* Vol 18, No 5, 1993, 1

Savaiano, DD et al. "Lactose Malabsorption from Yogurt, Pasteurized Yogurt, Sweet Acidophilus Milk, & Cultured Milk in Lactose-Deficient Individuals." *Am J Clin Nutr,* Vol 40, 1984, 1219–1223

Suarez, FL et al. "The Treatment of Lactose Intolerance." *Aliment Pharmacol Ther,* Vol 9, 1995, 589–597

Trapp, CL et al. "The Influence of Chronic Yogurt Consumption on Populations of Young & Elderly Adults." *Internatl J Immunother,* Vol 9, 1993, 53–64

Vanderhoff, J & R Young. "Role of Probiotics in the Management of Patients with Food Allergy." *Ann Allerg Asthma Immunol,* Vol 90, No 6, June 2003, S99–S103

Weizman, Z et al. "Effects of a Probiotic Infant Formula on Infections in Child Care Centers: Comparison of Two Probiotic Agents." *Pediat,* Vol 115, Jan 2005, 5–9

Chapter 9

Bankhead, CD. "Yogurt Wins Points in Test Against Recurring Vaginitis." *Med World News,* Oct 23, 1989, 31

Bruce, AW & G Reid. "Intravaginal Installation of Lactobaccilli for Prevention of Recurrent Urinary Tract Infections." *Can J Microbiol,* Vol 34, 1988, 339–343

Cadieux, P et al. "*Lactobacillus* Strains & Vaginal Ecology." Letter. *JAMA,* Vol 287, No 15, Apr 17, 2002, 1940–1941

Collin, EB & P Hardt. "Inhibition of *Candida albicans* by *Lactobacillus acidophilus.*" *J Dairy Sci,* Vol 63, 1980, 830–832

Conn, HO & MH Floch. "Effects of Lactose & *Lactobacillus acidophilus* on the Fecal Flora." *Am J Clin Nutr,* Vol 23, 1970, 1588–1594

"Daily Cup of 'Live' Yogurt Eases Infections." *Med Trib*, Mar 26, 1992, 25

Elmer, GW et al. "Biotherapeutic Agents: A Neglected Modality for the Treatment & Prevention of Selected Intestinal & Vaginal Infections." *JAMA*, Vol 275, No 11, Mar 20, 1995, 870–876

Eschenbach, DA et al. "Prevalence of Hydrogen Peroxide-Producing *Lactobacillus* Species in Normal Women & Women with Bacterial Vaginosis." *J Clin Microbiol*, Vol 27, No 2, 1989, 251–256

"Folk Remedy Seems to Help Fight Vaginal Yeast Infection." *NY Times*, Mar 10, 1992, C3

"Folk Therapy for Vaginitis Looking Good." Biomedicine. *Sci News*, Mar 7, 1992, 158

Friedlander, A et al. "*Lactobacillus acidophilus* & Vitamin B Complex in the Treatment of Vaginal Infection." *Panminerva Med*, Vol 28, No 1, 1986, 51–53

Gardiner, G et al. "Persistence of *Lactobacillus fermentum* RC-14 & *L. rhamnosus* GR-1, But Not *L. rhamnosus* GG in the Human Vagina as Randomly Amplified Polymorphis DNA (RAPD)." *Clin Diag Lab Immunol*, Vol 9, 2002, 92–96

Goldin, BR & SL Gorbach. "Alterations of the Intestinal Microflora by Diet, Oral Antibiotics, and *Lactobacillus:* Decreased Production of Free Amines from Aromatic Nitro Compounds, Azo Dyes, and Glucuronides." *J Natl Cancer Inst*, Vol 73, 1984, 689–695

Hallen, A. "Treatment of Bacterial Vaginosis with Lactobacilli." *Sex Trans Dis*, Vol 19, 1992, 146–148

Hillier, SI et al. "The Relationship of Hydrogen Peroxide Producing Lactobacilli to Bacterial Vaginosis & Genital Microflora in Pregnant Women." *Obstet Gynecol*, Vol 79, 1992, 369–373

——. "The Normal Vaginal Flora, H2O2-Producing Lactobacilli & Bacterial Vaginosis in Pregnant Women." *Clin Infect Dis*, Vol 16, 1993, Suppl 4, S273–S281

——. "Association between Bacterial Vaginosis & Preterm Delivery of a Low-Weight Infant." *N Engl J Med*, Vol 333, 1995, 1737–1742

Hilton, E et al. "Ingestion of Yogurt Containing *Lactobacillus acidophilus* as Prophylaxis for Candida Vaginitis." *Ann Intern Med*, Vol 116, No 5, Mar 1, 1992, 352–357

——. "*Lactobacillus* GG Vaginal Suppositories & Vaginitis." *J Clin Microbiol*, Vol 33, 1995, 1433

Hughes, VI & SL Hillier. "Microbiological Characteristics of *Lactobacillus* Products Used for Colonization of the Vagina." *Obstet Gynecol*, Vol 75, No 2, 1990, 244–248

Keating, H. "The Yogurt Controversy." *Cortlandt Forum*, June 1992, 212

Klebanoff, SJ et al. "Control of the Microbial Flora of the Vagina by H2O2-Generating Lactobacilli." *J Infect Dis*, Vol 164, 1991, 94–100

Kontiokari, T. "Randomized Trial of Cranberry-Lingonberry Juice & *Lactobacillus* GG Drink for the Prevention of Urogenital Probiotic Application." *Br Med J*, Vol 322, 2001, 157–173

Mardh, PA & LV Sultesz. "In Vitro Interaction between Lactobacilli & Other Microorganisms Occurring in the Vaginal Flora." *Scand J Infect Dis*, Vol 40, 1983, Suppl, 47–51

McFarland, LV & GW Welmer. "Biotherapeutic Agents: Past, Present, & Future." *Microecol Ther*, Vol 23, 1995, 46–73

McGroarty, JA. "Probiotic Use of Lactobacilli in the Human Female Urogenital Tract." *FEMS Immunol Med Microbiol*, Vol 6, 1993, 251–264

Reid, G et al. "Examination of Strains of Lactobacilli for Properties which May Influence Bacterial Interference in the Urinary Tract." *J Urol*, Vol 138, 1987, 330–335

——. "Is There a Role for Lactobacilli in Prevention of Urogenital & Intestinal Infections?" *Clin Microbiol Rev*, Vol 3, 1990, 335–344

——. "Influence of Three-day Antimicrobial Therapy & *Lactobacillus* Vaginal Suppositories on Recurrence of Urinary Tract Infections." *Clin Ther*, Vol 14, 1992, 11–16

——. "Implantation of *Lactobacillus casei* var *rhamnosus* into Vagina." *Lancet*, Vol 344, 1994, 1229

——. "Installation of *Lactobacillus* & Stimulation of Indigenous Organisms to Prevent Recurrence of Urinary Tract Infections." *Microecol Ther*, Vol 23, 1995, 32–45

——. "The Role of Lactobacilli in Preventing Urogenital & Intestinal Infections." *Interntl Dairy J*, Vol 8, 1998, 555–562

——. "Probiotic Agents to Protect the Urogenital Tract Against Infection." *Am J Clin Nutr*, 73, 2001 Suppl, 437S–443S

——. & AW Bruce. "Selection of *Lactobacillus* Strains for Urogenital Probiotic Applications." *J Infect Dis*, Vol 183, 2001 Suppl 1, S77–S80

——. "The Potential Role of Probiotics in Pediatric Urology." *J Urol*, Vol 168, Oct 2002, 1512–1517

Sanders, ME. "Healthful Attributes of Bacteria in Yogurt." *Contemp Nutr*, Vol 18, No 5, 1993, 1

Sandler, B. "*Lactobacillus* for Vulvovaginitis." *Lancet* II, 1979, 791–792

Sarra, PG & F Dellaglio. "Colonization of a Human Intestine by Four Different Genotypes of *Lactobacillus acidophilus.*" *Microbiol,* Vol 7, 1984, 331–339

Shalev, E et al. "Ingestion of Yogurt Containing *Lactobacillus acidophilus* Compared with Pasteurized Yogurt as Prophylaxis for Recurrent Candidal Vaginitis and Bacterial Vaginosis." *Arch Fam Med,* Vol 5, No 10, Nov-Dec 1996, 593–596

Sobel, JD. "Biotherapeutic Agents as Therapy for Vaginitis" in *Biotherapeutic Agents & Infectious Diseases,* GW Elmer, L McFarland, & C Surawcz, eds. Totowa, NJ: Humana Press, 1999

Will, TE. "*Lactobacillus* Overgrowth for Treatment of Moniliary Vulvaginitis." Letter. *Lancet* II, 1979, 482

Williams, A et al. "Weekly Treatment for Prophylaxis of Candida Vaginitis." *Presentation,* 7th Conference on Retroviruses & Opportunistic Infections. Foundation for Retrovirology & Human Health in Collaboration with Natl Inst Allerg Infect Dis & CDC. Jan 30–Feb 2, 2000

Wood, JR et al. "In Vitro Adherence of *Lactobacillus* Species to Vaginal Epithelial Cells." *Am J Obstet Gynecol,* Vol 153, 1985, 94–100

"Yogurt Found Immunogenic." *Med Trib,* Apr 23, 1991, 20

"Yogurt Ingestion Decreases Candidal Infection Threefold." *Am Med News,* Nov 1989, 4

"Yogurt's Active Bacteria Can Relieve Vaginal Infections." *Am Med News,* Dec 9, 1996, 32

Chapter 10

Bones

Aoe, S et al. "Controlled Trial of the Effects of Milk Basic Protein (MBP) Supplementation on Bone Metabolism in Healthy Adult Women." *Biosci Biotechnol Biochem,* Vol 65, 2001, 913–918

—— A Controlled Trial of the Effects of Milk Basic Protein (MBP) Supplementation on Bone Metabolism in Healthy Postmenopausal Women." *Osteopor Internatl,* Vol 16, 2005, 2123–2128

Heaney, RP et al. "Effect of Yogurt on a Urinary Marker of Bone Resorption on Postmenopausal Women." *J Am Diet Assoc,* Vol 102, No 11, Nov 2002, 1672–1674

Toba, Y et al. "Milk Basic Protein: A Novel Protective Function of Milk Against Osteoporosis." *Bones,* Vol 27, 2000, 403–408

—— "Milk Basic Protein Promotes Bone Formation & Suppresses Bone Resorption in Healthy Adult Men." *Biosci Biotechnol Biochem.* Vol 65, 2001, 1353–1357

Blood Pressure

"Fermented Milk Product Lowers Blood Pressure." *Nutr Reporter,* Apr 2006, 4

"Finnish Dairy Company Valio Has Launched a New Functional Cultured Milk with a Claim for Lowering Blood Pressure." Briefs. *Dietary Suppl Fd Label News,* Oct 18, 2000, 20

Hata, Y et al. "A Placebo-controlled Study of the Effect of Some Milk on Blood Pressure in Hypertensive Subjects." *Am J Clin Nutr,* Vol 64, 1996, 767–771

Jauhiainen, T et al. "Fermented Milk Product Lowers Blood Pressure." *Am J Hypertension,* Vol 18, 2005, 1600–1605

"Microbes for the Heart." *Prep Fds Nutra Sols,* Jan 2005, 22

Nakamura, Y et al. "Hypertensive Effect of Sour Milk & Peptides Isolated from It that Are Inhibitors to Angiotensin-1-converting Enzymes." *J Dairy Sci,* Vol 78, 1995, 1253–1257

——. "Decrease of Tissue Angiotensin-1-converting Enzyme Activity upon Feeding Sour Milk in Spontaneously Hypertensive Rats." *Biosci Biotech Biochem,* Vol 60, 1996, 488–489

Sawada, H et al. "Purification & Characterization of an Antihypertensive Compound from *Lactobacillus casei." Agric Biol Chem,* Vol 54, 1990, 3211–3219

Seppo, L et al. "A Fermented Milk High in Bioactive Peptides Has a Blood Pressure-Lowering Effect in Hypertensive Subjects." *Am J Clin Nutr,* Vol 77, Feb 2003, 326–330

Takano, T. "Milk Derived Peptides & Hypertension Reduction." *Internatl Dairy J,* Vol 8, 1998, 375–381

Cholesterol

Anderson, JW & SE Gilliland. "Effect of Fermented Milk (Yogurt) Containing *Lactobacillus acidophilus LI* on Serum Cholesterol in Hypercholesterolemic Humans." *J Am Coll Nutr,* Vol 18, 1999, 43–50

Brody, Jane E. "Study Hints that Yogurt May Reduce Cholesterol." Personal Health. *NY Times,* June 23, 1974

"Cholesterol Down—Not Up—with Milk & Yogurt." News & Notes. *Med Times,* May 1978, 3

"Claims Yogurt Reduces, Not Increases Cholesterol." *Dairy Record,* Mar 1978, 72

"Cultured Dairy Products Have Special Properties." *Fd Develop,* June 1981, 13

"Effects of Consuming Yogurts Prepared with Three Culture Strains on Human Serum Lipoproteins." *J Fd Sci,* July–Aug 1984, 1178–1181

Gilliland, SE et al. "An Assimilation of Cholesterol by *Lactobacillus acidophilus.*" *Appl Environ Microbiol,* Vol 49, 1985, 377–381

Gold, B & P Samuel. "Effect of Yogurt on Serum Cholesterol." *J Am Diet Assoc,* Vol 47, No 3, Sept 1965, 192–193

Hepner, B et al. "Hypocholesterolemic Effects of Yogurt & Milk." *Am J Clin Nutr,* Vol 32, 1979, 19–24

Kiebling, G et al. "Long-Term Consumption of Fermented Dairy Products Over 6 Months Increases HDL Cholesterol." *Eur J Clin Nutr,* Vol 56, Sept 2002, 843–849

Klaver, FAM & RV Meer. "The Assumed Assimilation of Cholesterol by Lactobacilli & *Bifidobacterium* Is Due to Their Bile Salt-Deconjugating Activity." *Appl Environ Microbiol,* Vol 59, 1993, 1120–1124

Mann, GV. "Studies of a Surfactant & Cholesteremia in the Masai." *Am J Clin Nutr,* Vol 27, 1974, 464–469

——. "The Masai, Milk & the Yogurt Factor: An Alternative Explanation." *Atherosclerosis,* Vol 29, 1978, 265

"Milk: A Cholesterol Fighter." Nutrition & Food, Research in Agriculture. *Penn State Progress Report,* Oct 1979, 5–6

Mital, RK & SK Garg. "Anticarcinogenic Hypocholesterolemic, and Antagonistic Activities of Lactic Acid." *Crit Rev Microbiol,* Vol 21, 1995, 175–214

Raloff, Janet. "*Acidophilus:* Milky Bane to Cholesterol?" *Sci News,* Vol 126, Aug 25, 1984, 118

Rasie, JL et al. "Assimilation of Cholesterol by Some Cultures of Lactic Acid Bacteria & Bifidobacteria." *Biotechnol Lett,* Vol 14, 1992, 39–44

Taylor, GR & CM Williams. "Effects of Probiotics & Prebiotics on Blood Lipids." *Br J Nutr,* Vol 80, 1998, Suppl 1, S225–S230

Tuhri, K et al. "Bifidobacteria Strain Behavior Toward Cholesterol: Coprecipitation with Bile Salts & Assimilation." *Curr Microbiol,* Vol 33, 1996, 187–193

Xiao, JZ et al. "Effects of Milk Products Fermented by *Bifidobacterium longum* on Blood Lipids in Rats & Healthy Adult Male Mice." *J Dairy Sci,* Vol 86, 2003, 2452–2461

"Yogurt Reduces Serum Cholesterol." *Dairy Field,* Oct 1979, 36

Eyes

Haworth, JC et al. "Effect of Galactose Toxicity on Growth of the Rat Fetus & Brain." *Pediat Res,* Vol 3, 1969, 441

Leger, RR. "Now Yogurt Is Struck by a Health Dispute: Tests on Rats Cited." *Wall St J,* June 15, 1970

Nagy, M. Questions & Answers. *JAMA*, Vol 217, No 8, Aug 23, 1971, 1113

Richter, CP & JR Duke. "Cataracts Produced in Rats by Yogurt." *Sci*, Vol 168, June 12, 1970, 1372–1374

——. "Yogurt-Induced Cataracts: Comments on Their Significance to Man." *JAMA*, 1970, Vol 214, 1878

Obesity

Hampton, Tracy. "Studies Link Intestinal Microbes with Obesity." *JAMA*, Vol 297, No 4, Jan 24–31, 2007, 353

Oral

Lichtenstein, J. *"Lactobacillus acidophilus* & Herpetic Gingivostomatis." *J Oral Ther Pharmacol*, Vol 1, 1964, 308

Nase, L et al. "Effect of Long-Term Consumption of a Probiotic Bacterium, *Lactobacillus rhamnosus* GG in Milk on Dental Caries & Caries Risk in Children." *Caries Res*, Vol 35, 2001, 412–420

Tumors

Adachi, S. "Lactic Acid Bacteria & the Control of Tumours" in *The Lactic Acid Bacteria in Health & Disease*. BJB Wood, ed. London, Eng: Elsevier Appl Sci, 1992, Vol 1, 233–261

"Anti-tumor Polysaccharides from *Lactobacillus*." *Agric Biol Chem*, Nov 1983, 1623–1625

Aso, Y & H Akazan. "Prophylactic Effect of a *Lactobacillus casei* Preparation on the Recurrence of Superficial Bladder Cancer." *Urol Internatl*, Vol 49, 1992, 125–129

Baricault, L et al. "Line of *HT-29*, a Cultured Human Colon Cancer Cell Line to Study the Effect of Fermented Milks on Colon Cancer Cell Growth & Differentiation." *Carcinogenesis*, Vol 16, 1995, 245–252

Bocci, Velio. "Tumor Therapy with Biological Response Modifiers: Why Is Progress Slow?" *EOS-J Immunol Immunopharmacol*, Vol 10, 1990, 79–82

Brudnak, MA. "Probiotics & Cancer." *Townsend Lett*, June 2002, 62–65

——. *The Probiotic Solution: Natures's Secret to Radiant Health*. St Paul, MN: Dragon Door Publ, 2003

Henriksson, R et al. "Effects of Active Addition of Bacterial Cultures in Fermented Milk in Patients with Chronic Bowel Discomfort Following Irradiation." *Support Care Cancer*, Vol 3, 1995, 81–83

Hill, M et al. "Bacteria & Etiology of Cancer of Large Bowel." *Lancet*, Jan 1971, 95–100

Hirayama, K & J Rafter. "The Role of Lactic Acid Bacteria in Colon Cancer Prevention: Mechanistic Considerations." *Antoine-Van-Leeuwenhoek*, Vol 76, 1999, 391–394

Nadathur, SR et al. "Lactic Acid Bacteria Produces Antimutagens in Yogurt." *Book of Abstracts*, Inst Fd Technol, paper #24C-2, 1994

——. "Isolation of Antimutagens from Yogurt." *Book of Abstracts*, Inst Fd Technol, paper #20–8, 1995

Rafter, JJ. "The Role of Lactic Acid Bacteria in Colon Cancer Prevention." *Scand J Gastroenterol*, Vol 30, 1995, 497–502

Rao, CV et al. "Prevention of Indices of Colon Carcinogenesis by the Probiotic *Lactobacillus acidophilus* NCFM in Rats." *Internatl J Oncol*, Vol 14, 1999, 939–944

Reddy, BS & A Rivenson. "Inhibitory Effect of *Bifidobacterium longum* on Colon, Mammary, and Liver Carcinogenesis Induced by Quinoline, a Food Mutagen." *Can Res*, Vol 53, 1993, 3914–3918

Renner, HW & R Munzner. "The Possible Role of Probiotics as Dietary Antimutagens." *Mutation Res*, Vol 262, 1991, 239–245

Salminen, E et al. "Preservation of Intestinal Integrity During Radiotherapy Using Live *Lactobacillus acidophilus* Cultures." *Chem Radiol*, Vol 39, 1988, 435–437

—— & E Salminen. "Clinical Uses of Probiotics for Stabilizing the Gut Mucosal Barrier: Successful Strains & Future Challenge." *Antoine van Leeuwenhoek*, Vol 70, 996, 347–358

Sessa, C. "Yogurt May Inhibit the Growth of Cancer." *Virginia-Pilot Tidewater Living*, Apr 30, 1975

Weaver-Missick, T. "A New Whey to Prevent Cancer?" *Agric Res*, Oct 2000, 10–11

Chapter 11

Almada, A. "Probiotics: Dead or Alive?" Appliance of Science. *Functional Fds Nutraceut*, May 2006, 62

Aston, A. "Bacteria: The Backbone of Fermentation." *Utah Sci*, Vol 63, 2006, 8–13

Bakalar, N. "A Bacterium that Improves Your Work Habits." Vital Signs. *NY Times*, Nov 15, 2005, F6

Benno, Y & T Mitsuoka. "Development of Intestinal Microflora in Human & Animals." *Bifidobact Microflora*, No 5, 1986, 13–25

Best, D. "Ride the Wave." *Prep Fds*, Aug 1997, 65

Boulloche, J et al. "Management of Acute Diarrhoea in Infants & Young Children:

Controlled Study of the Antidiarrhoeal Efficacy of Killed *L. acidophilus* (LB Strain) Versus a Placebo & a Reference Drug (loperamide)." *Ann Pediatr,* Vol 41, 1994, 457–463

Calder, P & S Kew. "The Immune System: A Target for Functional Foods?" *Br J Nutr,* Vol 88, 2002, Suppl 165–176

Colombel, JF et al. "Yogurt with *Bifidobacterium longum* Reduces Erythromycin-Induced Gastrointestinal Effects." *Lancet,* July 4, 1987, 43

Deguchi, Y et al. "Comparative Studies on Synthesis of Water-Soluble Vitamins Among Human Species of Bifidobacteria." *Agric Biol Chem,* Vol 49, No 1, 1985, 13–19

Duggan, C et al. "Protective Nutrients & Functional Foods for the Gastrointestinal Tract." *Am J Clin Nutr,* Vol 74, 2002, 789–808

Fujiwara, S et al. "Immunopotentiating Effects of *Bifidobacterium longum* SBT2928 (*BL 2928*) Showing Mitogenic Activity in Vitro." *J Japan Soc Nutr Fd Sci,* Vol 45, No 5, 1990, 327–333

Gorbach, SL. "The Discovery of *Lactobacillus* GG." *Nutr Today,* Vol 31, No 6, Nov–Dec 1990, Suppl S2–S4

Gorman, C. "Healthy Germs." *Time,* Dec 28, 1988, 197

Halpern, GH et al. "Treatment of Irritable Bowel Syndrome with Lacteol Fort: A Randomized, Double-Blind, Cross-Over Trial." *Am J Gastroenterol,* Vol 91, 1996, 1579-1585

Health & Nutritional Properties of Probiotics in Food, including Powder Milk with Five Lactic Acid Bacteria. Report of Joint FAO/WHO Expert Committees, 2001

Hoover, DG. "Bifidobacteria: Activity & Potential Benefits." *Fd Tech,* June 1993, 120–124

——. "The Probiotic Role of *Bifidobacterium* in the Human Intestinal System." *Book of Abstracts,* Inst Fd Technol, paper #2–3, 1995

Hotta, M et al. "Clinical Effects of *Bifidobacterium* Preparation on Pediatric Intractable Diarrhea." *Keio J Med,* Vol 36, No 12, 1987, 298–314

Ishibashi, N & S Shimamura. "Bifidobacteria: Research & Development in Japan." *Fd Tech,* Vol 47, No 6, June 1993, 126–128

Juntunen, M et al. "Adherence of Probiotic Bacteria to Human Intestinal Mucus in Healthy Infants & During Rotavirus Infection." *Clin Diagn Lab Immunol,* 2001

Kohwi, Y at al. "Antitumor & Immunological Adjuvant Effect of *Bifidobacterium infantis* in Mice." *Bifidobact Microflora,* No 1, 1982, 61–68

Miki, H. "Clinical Experiences of Bifidobacterial Dosage *BBG-02* on Chronic Constipation." *Jap Pharmacol Therapeut*, Vol 7, No 9, 1979, 2743–2747 (abstract)

Mitsuoka, T. "Bifidobacteria & Their Role in Human Health." *J Ind Microbiol*, No 6, 1990, 263–268 (abstract)

Modler, HW et al. "Bifidobacteria & Bifidogenic Factors." *Can Inst Fd Sci Technol J*, Vol 23, No 1, 1990, 29–41

Mulder, L. "Single Strains Vs Probiotic Stews." *Functional Fds Nutraceut*, Jan 2005, 36–37

Nakaya, R. "Role of *Bifidobacterium* in Enteric Infection." *Bifidobact Microflora*, Vol 3, No 1, 1984, 3–9

"New Cultures Produce 'Mild' Yougurt." *Fd Engineer*, Feb 1991, 71

Nishida, N et al. "Clinical & Bacteriological Studies for the Effect of Bifidobacterial Dosage *BBG-02* on Diarrhea & Constipation of Children." *Jap Pharmacol Therapeut*, Vol 7, No 4, 1979, 1032–1049

Okamura, N et al. "Interaction of *Shigella* with Bifidobacteria." *Bifidobact Microflora*, No 5, 1986, 51–55

"Out of the Refrigerator & Onto the Shelves." *Fd Quality*, Sept–Oct 2000, 38; 40

Owehand, AC et al. "The Mucous Binding of *Bifidobacterium lactis* BB-12 Is Enhanced in the Presence of *Lactobacillus* GG & *Lactobacillus debrueckii* spp. *bulgaricus*." Letter. *Appl Microbiol*, Vol 30, No 1, 2000, 103

Petesch, BL. "Lactic Acid Bacteria for Health." *Nutr in Complementary Care Newslett*. Practice Group of Am Diet Assoc, Vol 3, No 3, 2001, 53–54

Ray, C. "Beneficial Bacteria." Q & A. *NY Times*, Dec 5, 2006, D2

Sanders, ME. "Probiotics: Strains Matter." Food Science. *Functional Fds Nutraceut*, June 2007, 34–41

Sandine, WE. "Roles of Bifidobacteria & Lactobacilli in Human Health." *Contemp Nutr*, Vol 15, No 1, 1990, 1–2

Seki, M et al. "The Effect of *Bifidobacterium* Cultured Milk on the 'Regularity' Among an Aged Group." *J Jap Soc Fed Nutr*, Vol 31, No 4, 1978, 379–384

Shimek, JW et al. "Bifidobacteria Competition with *Clostridium perfringens* in Vivo & in Vitro." *Book of Abstracts*, Inst Fd Technol, paper #43–2, 1994

Simakachorn, N et al. "Clinical Evaluation of the Addition of Lyophilized Heat-Killed *Lactobacillus acidophilus* LB to Oral Rehydration Therapy in the Treatment of Acute Diarrhea in Children." *J Pediat Gastroenterol Nutr*, Vol 30, 2000, 68–72

"Specialty Dairy Additives." *Prep Fds*, Feb 1991, 78

Speck, ML. "Potential Benefits of Natural Lactic Acid Fermentation." *Dairy Field,* Jan 1980, 581

Tahvonen, R & Seppo S. "The Role of Functional Foods in Promoting Gut Health." Science Portal. *Functional Fds Nutraceut,* Apr 2006, 30–39

Tanaka, R & K Shimosaka. "Investigation of the Stool Frequency in Elderly Who Are Bedridden & Its Improvement by Ingesting Bifidus Yogurt." *Jap J Geriat,* Vol 19, No 6, 1982, 577–582

Teraguchi, S et al. "Vitamin Production of Bifidobacteria Originating from Human Intestine." *J Jap Soc Nutr Fd Sci.* Vol 37, No 2, 1984, 157–164

Timmerman, HM et al. "Monostrain, Multistrain, & Multispecies Probiotics—A Comparison of Functionality & Efficacy." *Internatl J Fd Microbiol,* Vol 96, 2004, 219–233

Tojo, M et al. "The Effects of *Bifidobacterium breve* Administration on *Campylobacter enteritis.*" *Acta Paediat Jap,* Vol 29, 1987, 160–167

Tomoda, T et al. "Effect of Yogurt & Yogurt Supplemented with *Bifidobacterium* and/or Lactulose in Healthy Persons: A Comparative Study." *Bifidobact Microflora,* Vol 10, No 2, 1991, 123–130

Tsuyuki, S et al. "Tumor-Suppressive Effect of a Cell Wall Preparation, *WPG,* from *Bifidobacterium infantis* in Germ-Free & Flora-Bearing Mice." *Bifidobact Microflora,* Vol 10, No 1, 1991, 43–52

Ueda, K. "Immunity Provided by Colonized Enteric Bacteria." *Bifidobact Microflora,* Vol 5, No 1, 1986, 67–72

Weiner, B & D Mills. "Enhancing Foods with Functional Genomics." *Fd Tech,* Vol 56, No 5, May 2002, 184–188

Wilkinson, S. "Making Food & Packaging Do More." Science & Technology. *C&EN,* Sept 20, 1999, 58–59

Xiao, SD et al. "Multicenter, Randomized, Controlled Trial of Heat-Killed *Lactobacillus* LB in Patients with Chronic Diarrhea." *Adv Ther,* Vol 20, 2003, 253–260

Yamazaki, S et al. "Protective Effect of *Bifidobacterium*-Monoassociation Against Lethal Activity of *Escherichia coli.*" *Bifidobact Microflora,* Vol 1, No 1, 1982, 55–59

——. "Immune Response of *Bifidobacterium*-Monoassociated Mice." *Bifidobact Microflora,* Vol 10, No 1, 1991, 19–31

Zimmer, C. "Bacterial Evolution in the Yogurt Ecosystem." *NY Times,* May 30, 2006, D3

Chapter 12

Frozen Yogurt

Alexander, RJ. "Moo-ving Toward Low-Calorie Dairy Products." *Fd Prod Design*, Apr 1997, 75–76; 79; 81–84; 87

"The Bright-Green Arithmetic of Frozen Yogurt: Location, Freezer Mix, Merchandising. Put Them All Together & You've Got Yourself a Gold Mine!" *Cooking for Profit*, Apr 1977, 30–32

Burros, M. "Frozen Yogurt: Tasty But No Health Food." *NY Times*, June 26, 1991, C1; C6

"Cashing in with the Soft Touch: Soft Serve Yogurt." *Fast Service*. Apr 1978, 41–43

"Composition for Stabilizing Soft Serve & Hard Frozen Yogurt." *Dairy Res Digest*, Vol 10, No 2, Feb 1980, 3

Dougherty, PH. "Frogurt—as American as Apple Pie." *NY Times*, Apr 6, 1977, D11

Durant, R. "Join the Yogurt Craze." *The Natl Dipper*, Apr 1989, 38

"FDA Clarifies Frozen Yogurt, Buttermilk Rule." *Dairy Record*, Sept 1977, 62

"Food Scientist Attacks Heat-Treated Yogurt." *Dairy Record*, May 1978, 48

Friedman, M. "Healthier Eating Trends Spark Frozen Yogurt Sales." *Dairy Fds*, June 1990, 27–28

"Frozen Yogurt Labeling Criticized." *Fd Chem News*, July 27, 1992, 49

"Frozen Yogurt May Get Own Standard." *Dairy Record*, Nov 1977, 46

"Frozen Yogurt Sales Expected to Rise." *Fd Engineer*, Nov 1989, 27

"Frozen Yogurt Should Not Contain Uncultured Milk." *Fd Chem News*, Sept 2, 1991, 36

"Frozen Yogurt Soft-Serve Unit." *Am Dairy Rev*, Dec 1977, 40

Grosser, V. "How to Make—and Sell—Hard-Frozen Yogurt." *Am Dairy Rev*, May 1978, 20; 22

"Heat Treatment of Cultured Dairy Products." *Dairy Res Digest*, Vol 10, No 1, Jan 1980, 1

Ifill, G. "Curdle Up a Little Closer: Yogurt Mine." *Boston Herald Am*, July 16, 1978, F1; F7

Kimbrell, W et al. "Mass Appeal: Frozen Yogurt Marketers May Not Have Standards of Identity, But that Isn't Stopping Consumers from Pushing Frozen Yogurt Sales to Record Heights." *Dairy Fds*, Vol 91, No 2, Feb 1990, 42–63

"Let Them Eat Yogurt." *Time*, Aug 30, 1976, 73

Maas, S. "Serving Up Profits! Here Are Some New & Innovative Ways to Use Soft-

Serve Machines for Merchandising & Profits, Capitalizing on the Growing Popularity of Frozen Soft-Serve Yogurt." Equipment. *Fd Service Marketing*, Apr 1977, 46–47

Martin, MC et al. "Lactose Digestion from Flavored & Frozen Yogurts, Ice Milk, & Ice Cream by Lactase-Deficient Persons." *Am J Clin Nutr*, Vol 46, 1987, 636–640

Meyer, A. "Will the Real Frozen Yogurt Please Stand Up." Food Business. *Prep Fds*, June 1989, 41–44

Pehanich, M. "The Yogurt Story: Health Gone Hollywood." *Prep Fds*, Oct 1984, 61–65

"Producers Cite 'Compelling' Need for Frozen Yogurt Standard." *Fd Chem News*, Oct 19, 1991, 20

Rane, PL. "Yogurt: Hot Stuff When Frozen." *Fd Service Marketing*, Oct 1976, 10

Sheraton, M. "But Is It Really Yogurt?" *NY Times*, Oct 23, 1976

——. "Putting Nature Back into the Frozen Yogurt." *NY Times*, Feb 12, 1977, C26

"Soft Serve Yogurt—the New Kid on the Block." *Fast Service*, Dec 1976, 21–27

"Stressing Health for Familiar Brand." *Pkging Digest*, June 2000, 30

Sugarman, C. "The Frozen Yogurt Trap: A Large Serving Topped with Candy Is No Caloric Bargain." *Wash Post Health*, Oct 16, 1990, 14

Tharp, BW. "Innovative Formulation for Frozen Yogurt." *Am Dairy Rev*, Ice Cream edition, Jan 1980, 14A–14E

"Two Years in the Making: Frozen Yogurt." *Am Dairy Rev*, Sept 1978, 64

Functional Foods

Anthony, M. "Digestive Health's New Phase." *Fd Proc Wellness Fds*, Aug 2006, 22

"Biopharmaceuticals." *Fd Engineer*, Dec 1989

"Cholesterol-Busting Yoghurt Drink." New Product. *Functional Fds Nutraceut*, Jan 2007, 43

Clemens, RA. "Friendly Bacteria: A Functional Food?" *Fd Tech*, Vol 55, No 1, Jan 2001, 27

Decker, KJ. "The Dominant Culture: Yogurt for the Masses." *Fd Prod Design*, Apr 2001, 89–106

Deis, RC. "Opportunities for Heart-Healthy Food." *Fd Prod Design*, Feb 2007, 63–75

Gerdes, S. "Yogurt: Enhancing a Superfood." *Fd Prod Design*, Mar 2007, 68–80

Klaenhammer, T. " The Probiotic Promise." *Prep Fds*, Mar 2001, 42–43

Kubomura, KR. " Yogurt Goes Nano-Platinum." *Prep Fds*, June 2007, 76

Nestle, M. *What to Eat*. NY: North Point Press, 2006, 473

"New Process Extends Yogurt Shelflife." *Fd Prod Design*, Dec 2006, 23

"A New Twist on Probiotics." New Products. *Prep Fds*, June 2000, 12–13

O'Donnell, CD. "The Biotics." *Prep Fds*, June 2007, 73–79

"Probiotic Drops for Infants & Older." *Functional Fds Nutraceut*, Dec 2006, 42

Roberts, WA. "Forecasting Food's Future." *Prep Fds*, Jan 2007, 23–28

Sanders, ME. "10 Myths About Probiotics." *Prep Fds*, July 2005, 67–73

Siuta-Cruce, P & J Goulet. "Improving Probiotic Survival Rate." *Fd Tech*, Oct 2001, 36–42

Toops, D. "Probiotic Gum to Debut." Healthbites. *Fd Proc Wellness Fds*, Dec 2006, 6

"Wellness Foods Trendsetters." *Fd Proc Wellness Fds*, Dec 2006, 24

Marketing

"Building Business on Milk & Honey." *Dairy Record*, Feb 1978, 52–54

"Dannon Milk Product." *Rest Bus*, May 1975, 45–46

"Dannon Opens First Yogurt Store." *Am Dairy J*, June 1975, 27

Elliott, RA. "Bostonians Enjoy Health Foods at Yogurt Yes!" *Am Dairy Rev*, Ice Cream edition. June 1978, 25E–26E

——. "Bel Air Yogurt Parlor Attracts Celebrities from Movies & TV." *Am Dairy Rev*, July 1978, 69–70

"Frozen Yogurt Stores: Will They Stay?" *Dairy Record*, July 1978, 68

Grant, HB. "Speaking for the Field." *Dairy Ice Cream Field*, Oct 1977, 38

Kanner, B. "On Madison Avenue: Cultural Revolution, the Yogurt Boom." *New York*, July 18, 1983, 14

Taylor, D. "Cultural Evolution: Are Probiotic Lactic Cultures Dairy's Seminal Step or Modest Marketing Ploy? *Fd Formul*, Oct 1995, 49–54

Vanderhoof, JA & RJ Young. "Current & Potential Uses of Probiotics. *Ann Allergy, Asthma, Immunol*, Vol 93, No 5, 2004, S533–S537

"Yogurt Eating Contests Emerge on College Scene." *Dairy Record*, June 1978, 92

Serving Size

Brody, JE. "Forget the Second Helpings: It's the First Ones that Supersize Your Waistline." Personal Health. *NY Times*, July 11, 2006, F7

Nestle, M. *Food Politics: How the Food Industry Influences Nutrition & Health*. Berkeley, CA: Univ Calif Press, 2002

Standards

"Borden on Yogurt: Labeling's the Issue; Not Live Culture Presence." *Dairy & Ice Cream Field*, Sept 1979, 12

Burros, M. "Does 'Yogurt' on the Label Make It So?" Eating Well, the Living Section, *NY Times*, Sept 19, 1990, C1

"Challenges 'Non-Yogurt' Yogurt." *Fd Proc*, Feb 1978, 96

"Doctors Recommend Yogurt with Live Active Cultures." *Fd Tech*, Jan 2002, 12

Dryer, J. "Consumers' Questions Need Answers." *Dairy Fds*, June 1990, 37

"FDA Sets Standards on Cultured Milk." *Fd Prod Devel*, Apr 1981, 8–10

Kazanas, JJ. "Preserve Yogurt's Identity." Letter. *Dairy & Ice Cream Field*, Sept 1977, 83

"Lawmakers Ask FDA to Consider Amendments to Yogurt Standards." *Diet Suppl Fd Label News*, Nov 8, 2000, 18

"National Nutritional Foods Association Sets *Acidophilus* Labeling." *Natl Fd Merchand*, Sept 1989, 6

"New Seal on Yogurt Packages Will Distinguish the Healthy Difference." Press Release. Natl Yogurt Assoc, Feb 25, 1993

"Production of Sterile Yoghurt." *Dairy Res Digest*, Vol 11, No 2, Feb 1981, 4

"Proposed Standards Would Require Special Labeling of Some Yogurts." *Fd Proc*, Sept 1977, 26

"Proposed Yogurt Standards Draw Reactions." *Dairy Record*, Jan 1978, 54

Reynes, C. "The Science of Probiotics." *Nutr for Optimal Health Newslett*, Vol 3, No 2, Spring 2006, 1–4

Sanders, ME. "10 Myths about Probiotics." *Prep Fds*, July 2005, 67–73

Speck, ML. "Heated Yogurt: Is It Still Yogurt?" *J Fd Protect*, Vol 40, No 12, Dec 1977, 863–865

Sugarman, C. "Sizing Up the Cultural Elite: Does the Yogurt Association's New Seal Really Help Consumers?" *Wash Post*, Mar 24, 1993, E1

"Urge Same Criteria for Yogurt, Milk." *Dairy Record*, Oct 1977, 50

"When Is Yogurt Yogurt?" *Dairy Record*, Nov 1977, 34–36

"Yogurt Association Petitions FDA on Yogurt Standard." News & Analysis: News of Societies & Association. *Fd Tech*, May 2000, 20

"Yogurt Is Only Yogurt with Live Bacteria." *Dairy Record*, July 1978, 68

"Yogurt Preservative Could Be Included in Label." *Dairy Record*, June 1978, 12

"Yogurtscam." *Rest Hosp*, Nov 1989, 36

"Yogurt Standard Imminent." *Dairy Record*, Oct 1978, 110–114

Yogurt

Brody, JE. "Make These Bacteria Go to Work for You." Personal Health. *NY Times*, Dec 25, 2001, F6

"Commercial Yogurts." *Dairy Record*, Mar 1980, 86–87

"Culturing Lies." *US News & World Report*, Dec 20, 1993

Decker, KJ. "The Dominant Culture: Yogurt for the Masses." *Fd Prod Design*, Apr 2001, 89–98; 101–106

Devero, JE. "Yogurt's Success in the United States." *Am Dairy Rev*, Milk Products Suppl, Feb 1979, 36A–36D

Dougherty, PH. "Yogurt from the Grant's Garden." *NY Times*, Sept 25, 1975

Elliott, RA. "Merchandising: Accent on Cultured Products." *Am Dairy Rev*, Sept 1978, 6

"Exotic Fermented Dairy Foods." *Dairy Res Digest*, Vol 8, No 1, Jan 1978, 2

"Fivefold Increase Predicted for Yogurt." *Dairy & Ice Cream Field*, Dec 1978, 15

"The Household Yogurt Market, Apr 1972–Mar 1973." Market Eco Res Div, United Dairy Ind Assoc, 1973

"Is 'Yogurt' Becoming a Household Word?" *Fd Proc*, Sept 1974, 45

Levitt, A. "Over 42.5 Billion Ounces Served—and Counting." *Dairy Fds*, Dec 1988, 58–61

Mann, J. "Kumiss Manufacturing Meeting Strong Consumer Demand for Yogurt." *Prep Fds*, Jan 1983, 78–80

McBean, LD. "Dairy Foods: Traditional & Emerging Health Benefits." *Dairy Council Digest*, Vol 69, No 5, 1998, 25–30

Nestle, M. *What to Eat*. NY: North Point Press, 2006, 99–107

Nielsen, VH. "Outlook for Building Consumer Acceptance for Cultured Products." *Am Dairy Rev*, Jan 1976

Quackenbush, GG. "The Sales Potential for Cultured Dairy Products." *Am Dairy Rev*, Milk Products Suppl, Jan 1976, 18B

——. "More Americans Liking Yogurt More & More." *Dairy Record*, Feb 1978, 47–50

"Sales of Frozen Yogurt Continue to Rise." *Fd Engineer*, Jan 1990, 38

Starling, S. "Probiotic Culture Developing Beyond Yoghurt." *Functional Fds Nutraceut*, Nov 2005, 6

"U.S. Wolfing Yogurt by the Ton." *C&EN*, Oct 1, 1973, 48

Wagner, JN. "Who's Dunking Yogurt?" *Fd Engineer*, Sept 1981, 108–109

Watt, JW. "Cultured Dairy Products." Letter. *Am Dairy Rev*, Oct 20, 1975

Williams, RD. "Yogurt: The Curds & Whey to Health?" *FDA Consumer*, June 1992, 27–33

"Yogurt: A Compositional Survey." *Dairy Record*, Sept 1979, 100

"Yogurt Consumption Booms—Up 3,410%." *Dairy Record*, Sept 1977, 60–62

"Yogurt Forms & Flavors Boom: Forecast $600 Million Sales for 1978." *Fd Proc*, Apr 1977, 66–69

"Yogurt's Fast Growth Per Capita Consumption." Bar Graph. *Pkging*, Apr 1986, 3

Chapter 13

Acidophilus

"Acidophilus Milk." Milk Information Sheet. Chicago, IL: Natl Dairy Council, 1971

"'Bugged' Milk Not Therapeutic." *Med World News*, Jan 10, 1977, 10

"Case for Acidophilus Milk Not Proved, Says NY State." *Consumer Repts*, Mar 1977, 167

"Crowley Foods Says New Milk Product Has Health Benefits." *Wall St J*, Mar 16, 1976, 14

"Exclusive Agent Named for Sweet Acidophilus Milk Cultures." *Prep Fds*, Apr 1985, 42

"Food for Thought—Sweet Acidophilus Brand Milk Nu-Trish." *Dairy Record*, Jan 1978, 9

"Idlenot Brings You the First New Milk Since 1944." Brochure. Idlenot Dairy, 1976

Key, D. "*Lactobacillus acidophilus* and Health." *Brattleboro Reformer*, (Brattleboro, VT), July 28, 1978, 7

"L.I. Milk Company Agrees to End Therapeutic Claim for Acidophilus Product." *NY Times*, Dec 6, 1976, C41

"Many Dairies Are Selling New Sweet Acidophilus Milk." *Am Dairy Rev*, July 1976, 30

Mayer, J & J Dwyer. "Sweet Acidophilus: Risks & Benefits." *Daily News*, Dec 29, 1976

Mustapha, A et al. "Improvement of Lactose Digestion by Humans Following Ingestion of Unfermented Acidophilus Milk: Influences of Bile Sensitivity, Lactose Transport, and Acid Tolerance of *Lactobacillus acidophilus*." *J Dairy Sci*, Vol 80, 1997, 1537–1545

"New Acidophilus Milk Is Not Sour Milk." *NY Times*, Nov 14, 1976, 60

"New Method of Acidophilus Milk Manufacture." *Dairy Res Digest*, (Part 1) Vol 8, No 4, Apr 1978, 3; (Part 2) Vol 8, No 11, Nov 1978, 3

"New N.C. State Process Enhances Milk's Value." *Transylvania Times* (Brevard, NC), Jan 2, 1975

Nielsen, VH. "Sources of Protein Predominant Topic at ADSA Meeting." *Am Dairy Rev*. Ice Cream Suppl, acidophilus milk, Oct 1974, 20

Pearce, J. "Milk No Longer a Sacred Cow." *Fam Health*, Aug 1978, 28–29

Saltzman, JR et al. "A Randomized Trial of *Lactobacillus acidophilus* BG2FQ4 to Treat Lactose Intolerance." *Am J Clin Nutr*, Vol 69, 1999, 40–46

Speck, ML. "The Development of Sweet Acidophilus Milk." *Dairy & Ice Cream Field*, Mar 1978, 70A–70D

"Sweet Milk with Good Bugs Nutrition." *Med World News*, Oct 18, 1976, 7–8

"Sweet Success of Sweet Acidophilus." News Feature. *Dairy Record*, Mar 1978, 42–43: 46

Zamula, E. "Beyond Yogurt: Milking the Public's Taste for Exotic Health Foods." *FDA Consumer*, Nov 1986, 12–15

Buttermilk

Andres, C. "Culture for Buttermilk Provides Operating Efficiencies." *Fd Proc*, May 1983, 46

Een, AJ. "Buttermilk in the 1920s: The Memories Linger." Dairy Diary. *Dairy Record*, Apr 1980, 112

Filipic, M. "Thank Fermentation for Buttermilk." Chow Line Release. Wooster, OH: Ohio State Univ, Dec 25, 2005

Hunter, BT. *Consumer Beware! Your Food & What's Been Done to It*. NY: Simon & Schuster, 1971, 240

Jones, ID. "Effects of Processing by Fermentation on Nutrients" in *Nutritional Evaluation of Food Processing*, Robert S. Harris & Endel Karmas, eds. Westport, CT: Avi Publ Co, 1975, Ch 12, 329

Kristofferson, T & IA Gould. "Manufacturing Practices for Cultured Buttermilk in Ohio Dairy Plants." *J Dairy Sci*, Vol 49, 1966, 690–693

McGee, C. *"On Food & Cooking: The Science & Lore of the Kitchen*. NY: Charles Scribner's Sons, 1984, 34–35

"Nutrition." *Wash Post*, June 17, 1992, E12

Olson, NF. "Benefitting from Lactic Bacteria." *Dairy Field*, Dec 1979, 99A

"On the Fridge." *Wash Post,* Aug 23, 1989, E3

"Quality of Commercial Buttermilk." *Dairy Record,* Dec 1979, 121

Squires, S. "Buttermilk Is Not what It Sounds Like." *Wash Post Health,* Mar 2, 1993, 16

"What is Buttermilk?" *Am Health,* Mar 1991, 10

"What's Old Fashioned Is New Again." On the Shelf. *Prep Fds Wellness Fds,* Oct 2004, 8

Kefir

Claiborne, C. Q & A, *NY Times,* Jan 28, 1983, C10

Damn, H. "Preparation of Kefir, Yoghurt & Acidophilus Milk." *Apoth Ztg,* Vol 44, 1929, 1127–1130

Deis, RC. "New Directions for Cultured Dairy Products." *Fd Prod Design,* Mar 2000, 84–99

"Directions for Making Kefir Fermented Milk." Agric Res Admin, Bur Dairy Ind, USDA, No 58, Nov 1947

Farnsworth, ER. "Kefir: From Folklore to Regulatory Approval." *J Nutraceut Functional Med Fd,* No 1, 1999, 57–68

——. "Kefir: A Complex Probiotic." *Fd Sci Technol Bull.* No 2, 2005, 1–17

Foster, K. "Vitamin Content of Kefir." *Biochem Z,* 1931, 238

Furukawa, N et al. "Effects of Fermented Milk on the Delayed-Type Hypersensitivity Response & Survival Day in Mice Bearing Meth-A." *Anim Sci Technol,* Vol 62, 1991, 579–585 (abstract)

Ginsberg, AS. "Chemical Processes in the Fermentation of Kumiss & Kefir." *Biochem Z.* Vol 30, 1911, 1–38

Hertzler, SR & SM Claney. "Kefir Improves Lactose Digestion & Tolerance in Adults with Lactose Maldigestion." *J Am Diet Assoc,* Vol 103, No 5, May 2003, 582–588

Karlin R. "Enrichment of Kefir in Vitamin B12 through Microbial Association of *Propionibacterium shermanii.*" *Compt Rend Soc Biol,* Vol 155, 1961, 1309–1313, abstract in *Chem Abstracts,* Vol 56, No 8, 1962, 9171f

"Kefir." *Am Dairy Rev,* Oct 1978, 52, 54

Kneifel, W & HK Mayer. "Vitamin Profiles of Kefirs Made from Milks of Different Species." *Internatl J Fd Sci Technol,* Vol 26, 1991, 423–428

Kosikowski, F. *Care & Drying of Kefir Grains.* Dept Dairy & Fd Sci, Cornell Univ, undated

Kroger, M. "Kefir." *Cult Dairy Prods*, Vol 28, 1993, 26; 28–29

Kubo, M et al. "Pharmacological Study of Kefir: A Fermented Milk Product in Caucasus: on Antitumor Activity." *Yakugaku Zasshi*, Vol 112, 1992, 489–495 (abstract)

Mainville, I et al. "Polyphasic Characteristics of the Lactic Acid Bacteria in Kefir." *Syst Appl Microbiol*, Vol 29, 2006, 59–68

Montery, A. "Manufacture of Fermented Beverages from Milk." *Lait*, Vol 17, 1937, 545–549

Murofushi, M et al. "Effect on Orally Administered Polysaccharide from Kefir Grain on Delayed-Type Hypersensitivity & Tumor Growth in Rats." *Jap J Med Sci Biol*, Vol 36, 1983, 49–53 (abstract)

——. "Immunopotentiative Effect of Polysaccharide from Kefir Grain KGF-C Administered Orally in Mice." *Immunopharmacol*, Vol 12, 1986, 29–35 (abstract)

Roberts, Jr, WA. "Claiming a Function." New Product Trends. *Prep Fds*, Sept 2006, 11–19

Rosell, JM. "Yoghourt & Kefir in Their Relation to Health & Therapeutics." Historical Notes. *Can Med Assoc J*, Vol 26, 1932, 341–345

——. "Manufacturing of Popular European Special Milks: Kefir, Yoghourt, and Kumiss." *Milk Dealer*, Vol 24, No 7, 1935, 41–44

——. "Yoghourt & Kefir & Their Relation to Health & Therapeutics." *Can Med Assoc J. Child Family Digest*. Vol 18, Jan–Feb 1959, 85

Shiomi, M et al. "Antitumor Activity in Mice of Orally Administered Polysaccharide from Kefir Grains." *Jap J Med Sci Biol*, Vol 35, 1982, 75–80 (abstract)

Vujicic, JF et al. "Assimilation of Cholesterol in Milk by Kefir Cultures." *Biotechnol Lett*, Vol 14, 1992, 847–850

Wildman, RE, ed. *Handbook of Nutraceuticals & Functional Foods*. 2nd ed. Boca Raton, FL: CRC Press, 2006, 344–346

Kumiss and Other Traditional Fermented Dairy Products

"Egyptian Fresh Fermented Milk Products." *Dairy Res Digest*, Vol 14, No 8, Apr 1984, 3

Jones, ID. "Effects of Processing by Fermentation of Nutrients" in *Nutritional Evaluation of Food Processing*, Robert S. Harris & Endel Karmas, eds. 2nd ed. Westport, CT: Avi Publ, 1975, Ch 12, 324–332

Pulytov, RP et al. "Vitamin B12 in Mare's Milk & in Koumiss *Sb Tr.Us. Nauchn-Issled Inst Tuberkuleza*," Vol 5, 1961, 186–188, (abstract) in *Chemical Abstracts*, Vol 59, No 12, Dec 9, 1963

"Quarg Gains Popularity in Europe, Opportunity Likened to Yogurt." Product Development News. *Fd Prod Devel*, Mar 1980, 12

"Ultrafiltration Is the Key in New Junket-Making Process (Ymer)." *Fd Engineer*, Mar 1976, 84–85

Tannahill, R. *Food in History*. NY: Stein & Day, 1973, 134–136

Sour Cream

Burros, M. "Finding Crème Fraîche." *NY Times*, July 24, 1982, 46

McGee, H. *"On Food & Cooking: The Science & Lore of the Kitchen*. NY: Scribner's Sons, 1984, 35–36

"Sour Cream: How to Prepare & Use It at Home." Leaflet No 213, USDA, Oct 1941

"Sour Product Enjoys Sweet Success." *Battelle Today*, No 3, Feb 1977, 1

Tannahill, R. *Food in History*. NY: Stein & Day, 1973

Chapter 14

Pickles

Camillo, LJ et al. "An Analytical Study of Cucumbers & Cucumber Pickles." *Fd Res*, No 7, 1942, 339–352

Cheigh, HS & KY Park. "Biochemical, Microbiological & Nutritional Aspects of Kimchi (Korean Fermented Vegetable Products)." *Crit Rev Fd Sci Nutr*, Vol 34, 1994, 175–203

Chun, K. "Kimchi." *Fd Arts*, Jan–Feb 1998, 66–71

Jones, I. "Effects of Processing by Fermentation on Nutrients" in *Nutritional Evaluation of Food Processing*, 2nd ed., Robert S Harris & Endel Karmas, eds, Westport, CT: Avi Publ, 1975, 332–333

"Space Kimchi." *Sci*, May 5, 2006, 667

Uhl, S. "Pickle in the Middle." *Fd Prod Design*, Nov 2000, 164

Sauerkraut

Bash, W. "Why Is Sauerkraut Sour? Smart Stuff with Twig Walkingstick." *Release*, Columbus, OH: Ohio State Univ, Dec 27, 1998

Cowan, T. "Lacto-Fermentation." *Aurum Update*, Winter 1998, 2–3

McGee, H. *On Food & Cooking: The Science & Lore of the Kitchen*. NY: Charles Scribner's Sons, 1984, 173

Pederson, CS et al. "Vitamin C Content of Sauerkraut." *Fd Res*, No 4, 1939, 31–45

——. "The Ascorbic Acid Content of Sauerkraut." *Fd Tech*, No 10, Oct 1956, 365–367

—— & MM Albury. *The Sauerkraut Fermentation*. NY State Agr Exp Sta Bull, No 824, 1969

Raloff, J. "Fighting Cancer from the Cabbage Patch." *Sci News*, Apr 23, 2000, 198

Reddy, NR et al. *Legume-Based Fermented Foods*. Boca Raton, FL: CRC Press, 1986

Vegetables

Gammack, DB. "Nutrition & Toxicology of Fermented Foods" in *Nutritional & Toxicological Aspects of Food Processing*. R Walker & E Quattrucci, eds. NY: Taylor & Francis, 1988, 231–237

Harris, LJ. "The Microbiology of Vegetable Fermentations" in *Microbiology of Fermented Foods*, BJB Wood, ed. London, Eng: Blackie Academic & Professional Tomson Sci, 1998, 45–72

Jones, ID. "Fermented Vegetable Products" in *Nutritional Evaluation of Food Processing*, Robert S Harris & Endel Karmas, eds, Westport, CT: Avi Publ, 1975, 2nd ed. 324–354

Chapter 15

Miso

Shurtleff, W & A Aoyagi. *The Book of Miso: Food for Mankind*. NY: Ballantine, 1976, rev ed

Thornton, M. "Australia's Food Regulator Warns of Cancer-Causing Soy Sauces." *Fd Chem News*, June 10, 2002, 19

Natto

Elder, SJ et al. "Vitamin K Contents of Meat, Dairy & Fast Food in the U.S. Diet." *J Agric Fd Chem*, Vol 54, 2006, 463–467

Runestad, T. "K: The Latest Addition to the Vitamin Alphabet Soup." Internatl Market, *Functional Fds Nutraceut*, May 2007, 6

Sano, T. "Feeding Studies with Fermented Soy Products (Natto & Miso)," in Meeting Protein Needs of Infants & Children. Wash, DC: Natl Acad Scs/Natl Res Council, Publ 843, 1961

Shoyu

Ferretti, F. "Imperial Shoyu: The World's Most Exclusive Soy Sauce." *Fd Arts*, Apr 2001, 175–178

Soybean

Daniel, KT. *The Whole Soy Story: The Dark Side of America's Favorite Health Food*, Wash, DC: New Trends Publ, 2005

Prasad, AS, ed. *Zinc Metabolism*. Springfield, IL: Charles C Thomas, 1966, 207

Reddy, NR, MD Pierson & DK Salunkhe, eds. *Legume-Based Fermented Foods*. Boca Raton, FL: CRC Press, 1986

"Taking the Wind Out of Beans." Sci & Tech Concentrate. *C&EN*, July 7, 2003, 17

Tempeh

Steinkraus, KH et al. "Studies on Tempeh: An Indonesian Fermented Soybean Food." *Fd Res*, Vol 25, 1960, 777–788

——. "A Pilot-Plant Process for the Production of Dehydrated Tempeh." *Fd Tech*, Vol 19, Jan 1965, 63–68

Tofu

Meyers, H et al. "Foodborne Botulism from Home-Prepared Fermented Tofu—California 2006." *CDC's MMWR*, Vol 56, No 5, Feb 9, 2007, 96–97

Miller, CD et al. "Retention of Nutrients in Commercially Prepared Soybean Curd." *Fd Res*, Vol 17, 1952, 261–267

Shurtleff, W & A Aoyagi. *The Book of Tofu*. NY: Ballantine, 1979

Chapter 16

"Healthful Fermented Barley." *Fd Prod Design*, Sept 2006, 121

Hughes, K. "Healthy Bread Flavors." *Prep Fds*, Apr 2007, 73

Hunter, BT. *The Natural Foods Cookbook*. NY: Simon & Schuster, 1961, 168

——. *The Natural Foods Primer: Help for the Bewildered Beginner*. NY: Simon & Schuster, 1972, 118; 132–137

Jones, ID. "Effects of Processing by Fermentation of Nutrients" in *Nutritional Evaluation of Food Processing*, Robert S. Harris & Endel Karmas, eds, Westport, CT: Avi, 1975, 2nd ed, 338

McGee, C. *On Food & Cooking: The Science & Lore of the Kitchen*. NY: Charles Scribner's Sons, 1984, 275; 313

"A Natural Start to a Natural Label." *Prep Fds Nutra Sols*, Sept 2006, NS7

Oberleas, D et al. "The Availability of Zinc from Foodstuffs" in *Zinc Metabolism*, Ananda S. Prasad, ed, Springfield, IL: Charles C Thomas, 1966, 225–238

Rajalakshmi, R & K Vanaja. "Chemical & Biological Evaluation of the Effects of Fermentation on the Nutritive Value of Foods Prepared from Rice & Grains." *Br J Nutr,* Vol 21, 1967, 467–472

Sanchez-Fernandez, CG & LL McKay. "Microbial Antagonism of *Agrobacterium azotophilum* from Pozol, an Indigenous Fermented Food from Mexico." *Book of Abstracts,* Inst Fd Technol, 1994, abstract No 55–1

Tannahill, R. *Food in History.* NY: Stein & Day, 1973, 66–69

Welch, H. "Ingredient of the Month: Kombucha." *Functional Fds Nutraceut,* July 2005, 8

Appendix A: Probiotics as Dietary Supplements

Dash, SK. "Selection Criteria for Probiotic Supplements." *Townsend Lett Doctors Patients,* Feb–Mar 2003, 99–101

Guamer, F & GF Schaafsma. "Probiotics." *Internatl J Fd Microbiol,* Vol 39, 1998, 237–238

Hamilton-Miller, JMT et al. "Probiotic Remedies Are Not What They Seem." Letter. *Br Med J,* Vol 312, No 7022, Jan 6, 1996, 55–56

"An Introduction to Probiotics." Natl Center Complement Alternat Med, NIH, Jan 2007, 1–6

Klaenhammer, TR & MJ Kullen. "Selection & Design of Probiotics." *J Fd Microbiol,* Vol 50, 1999, 45–57

——. "Probiotic Bacteria: Today & Tomorrow." *J Nutr,* Vol 130, Suppl, 415S–416S

——. "The Probiotic Promise." *Prep Fds Nutra Sols,* Mar 2001, 42–44

Nestle, Marion. *What to Eat.* NY: North Point Press, 2006, 473

"A New Twist on Probiotics." New Products. *Prep Fds,* June 2000, 12–13

"Probiotic Drops for Infants & Older." *Functional Fds Nutraceut,* Dec 2006, 42

Sheklke, K. "Gut News." *Fd Proc,* July 2003, 36–38

"That 'Gut' Feeling." *Prep Fds Nutra Sols,* Sept 2006, NS16

Toops, D. "Probiotic Gum to Debut." Health Bites. *Prep Fds Wellness Fds,* Dec 2006

Vogel, G. "Deaths Prompt a Review of Experimental Probiotic Therapy." Sci, Vol 319, Feb 1, 2008, 557

Appendix B: Bioactive Probiotic Components in Milk

Conjugated Linoleic Acid

Daiman, TR et al. "Conjugated Linoleic Acid Content of Milk from Cows Fed Different Diets." *J Dairy Sci,* Vol 82, No 10, 1999, 146–156

Kelly, ML et al. "Effect of Intake of Pasture and Concentrations of Conjugated Linoleic Acid in Milk of Lactating Cows." *J Dairy Sci,* Vol 81, No 6, 1998, 1630

Lactoferrin

Bellamy, W et al. "Identification of the Bactericidal Domain of Lactoferrin." *J Appl Bacteriol,* Vol 73, 1992, 472–479

"Biopharmaceuticals." *Fd Engineer,* Dec 1989, 58

Burrington, KJ. "Dairy Ingredients for Health." *Fd Prod Design,* Oct 1999, 53–56

"Dutch Company Develops Lactoferrin." *Fd Formulat,* Jan 1996, 29

Katz, F. "Cellular Research Defines Bioactive Components in Milk." *Fd Tech,* Vol 51, No 8, Aug 1997, 91–92

Labell, F. "Milk Proteins Protect Health." *Prep Fds,* July 2000, 77

O'Donnell, CD. "A Globe-Trotting Nutritional." *Prep Fds Nutra Sols,* June 2000, NS3

"A Powerful Bioactive Protein: Bovine Lactoferrin." *Fd Prod Design,* July 1998, 113

Reymeyer, JJ. "Milk Therapy: Breast Milk Could Be a Tonic for Adults." *Sci News,* Dec 9, 2006, 376–378

Seppa, N. "Gene Might Underlie Travelers' Diarrhea." *Sci News,* Oct 28, 2006, 286

"Utilizing Lactoferrin." *Prep Fds Nutra Sols,* July 2006, NS8

Whey

Burrington, KJ. "Dairy Ingredients for Health." *Fd Prod Design.* Oct 1999, 39–61

Carroll, M. "Natural Preservative for Safer Food, Less Waste." News Release, No 63, Columbus, OH: Ohio State Univ, Dec 31, 1992

Child, R. "The Wheys of Weight Loss." *Functional Fds Nutraceut,* Mar 2005, 62–71

Ennen, S. "Studies Suggest Broad Advantages for Whey." *Fd Proc,* July 2001, 80

Haines, B. "The Power of Protein." *Functional Fds Nutraceut,* May 2005, 50;52

"Hydrolyzed Whey Protein Isolate Benefits." *Fd Prod Design,* Nov 2002, 26

"In the Whey." *Prep Fds,* Nov 2001, 19

Karp, NRJ. "Electro-Dialyzed Whey-Based Foods for Use in Chronic Uremia." *J Am Diet Assoc,* Vol 59, 1971, 568–571

O'Neil, J. "New Clues on Relief for Colicky Infants." Vital Signs. *NY Times,* Jan 2, 2001, D6

"Parting of the Whey." *Fd Prod Design,* Suppl on Dairy Fds, June 2001, unpaginated

Schultz, M. "A Tale of Two Proteins." *Fd Prod Design,* Suppl, Aug 2005, unpaginated

"Study to Cut Waste Whey." Service, USDA's Report to Consumers, press release, May 1971, 3

"Whey: Now an Asset." *Agric Res*, Aug 1967, 7

Zinci, T. "Whey Fires Functional Sales." Foods of Tomorrow: Whey. *Fd Proc*, Aug 2000, 70–71

Appendix C: Colostrum

"Antibody-Rich Protein Ingredient." *Prep Fds*, Sept 1999, 88

Bitzan, MM et al. "Inhibition of *Helicobacter pylori* & *Helicobacter mustelac* Binding to Lipid Receptors by Bovine Colostrum." *J Infect Dis*, Vol 177, Apr 1998, 955–961

"Colostrum-Derived Immune Components Fight Pathogens, Help GI Tract." Products & Technologies. *Fd Tech*, June 1999, 164

Cutler, E. *Winning the War Against Immune Disorders & Allergies*. Florence, KY: Delmar Thomson Learning, 1998

Davidson, GP. "Passive Immunization of Children with Bovine Colostrum-Containing Antibodies to Human Rotavirus." *Lancet* II, 1989, 709–712

Durgan, A. "Colostrum for Immunity." Supplement Brief. *Natural Health*, June 2000, 43

Holt, S. "Colostrum as a Dietary Supplement: Focus on Transfer Factor." *Alternat Complement Therap*, Vol 4, No 4, Aug 1998, 276–283

Nitsch, A & FP Nitsch. "The Clinical Use of Bovine Colostrum." *J Orthomol Med*, Vol 13, No 2, 2nd Quarter 1998, 110–118

Wilson, J. "Immune System Breakthrough: Colostrum." *J Longevity*, Vol 4, No 2, 1998

Index

About the Author

Beatrice Trum Hunter has written nearly thirty books on food issues, including *Consumer Beware: Your Food & What's Been Done to It* (Simon & Schuster, 1971), *The Mirage of Safety: Food Additives and Public Policy* (Charles Scribner's Sons, 1975), *Food & Your Health* (Basic Health, 2003), *A Whole Foods Primer* (Basic Health, 2007), and *The Sweetener Trap & How to Avoid It* (Basic Health, 2008). As food editor for more than twenty years at *Consumers' Research Magazine*, her monthly columns and feature articles brought cutting-edge issues before general recognition.

Hunter has received many awards and recognitions for her work. The International Academy of Preventive Medicine made her an Honorary Fellow. Other honorary memberships include the American Academy of Environmental Medicine, the Price-Pottenger Nutrition Foundation, the Weston A. Price Foundation, and the Nutrition for Optimal Health Association. She received the prestigious Jonathan Forman Award for outstanding contributions to the field of environmental medicine, was honored by the International College of Applied Nutrition, and was recipient of the President's Award for the National Nutritional Foods Association.